Dedicated to Stephanie, Alexa,
Eleni, and Mary Cocores,
Richard Saleeby, George Balsama, Ph.D.,
and Richard DeSimone
for providing the inspiration
to write this book.

CONTENTS

Acknowledgements . . . 3

Preface . . . 4

Chapter One: How Healthy Brain Cells Help Us Learn . . . 6

Chapter Two: Brain Cells Work for *BrightFoods*:
How Food Affects Learning, Memory, Mood, and Performance . . . 11

Chapter Three: Brighten Your Mind: Reduce Brain Rust . . . 26

Chapter Four: Vital Oils Expand Brain Networking and Memory . . . 40

Chapter Five: Smart Proteins: Instant Messengers on the Brain-Wide Web . . . 53

Chapter Six: Slowly Absorbed Glucose: High-Speed Access to Well-Being . . . 65

Chapter Seven: Toxins: Part of a Modern Diet . . . 77

Chapter Eight: Immaterial Enrichment for the Brain and Mind . . . 95

Chapter Nine: *BrightFoods* Sample Menus and Recipes . . . 110

Chapter Ten: *BrightFoods* Programs from Text to Table . . . 147

Appendix I: *BrightFoods* Pyramid . . . 151

Appendix II: Fish School . . . 152

Appendix III: Glucose Absorption Rate of Various Foods . . . 155

Appendix IV: Drinking and Bottled Water Contaminants . . . 158

Appendix V: The Roots of *BrightFoods* Eating . . . 159

Medical Journal Sources . . . 161

Internet Addresses . . . 199

Index . . . 200

About the Author . . . 207

ACKNOWLEDGEMENTS

I would like to thank my mentors: Robert K. Davies, M.D.; Mark S. Gold, M.D.; A. Carter Pottash, M.D.; Donald R. Sweeney, M.D., Ph.D.; Javed Iqbal, M.D.; and Peter S. Mueller, M.D. They taught me that medical discoveries are made by carefully listening to patients.

Research assistants for an earlier version of this book were Eleni Cocores (additives), Alexa Cocores (lycopene and pesticide residue assays), Stephanie Cocores (mercury in fish assays), Chef Adam Wertheimer (culinary consultant), and Joyce Wertheimer, Ph.D., (antioxidant teas). The independent editor for a book proposal of the earlier version was Susan A. Schwartz, which was taken to a crowded market by the Jeff Herman Literary Agency.

Special thanks to Roxiticus Ventures for suggesting the book's format, Jen Zuccolo for technical support, and Dale Calvert for design and marketing suggestions.

Finally, I am most grateful to the nutrition experts and physicians who served as medical editors, and for the editorial assistance of Cindy Schweich Handler.

PREFACE

Americans are always on the move. We're the world's most productive employees, working ever-longer hours; when we're not in the office, we're commuting, traveling, multitasking, and chauffeuring our kids, who are themselves studying during ever-lengthening school days, learning to be prepared for the global marketplace.

Living in our culture these days takes a tremendous amount of focus. Unfortunately, at a time when so much is required of us, this seems to be exactly what we're lacking. Too often, we space out by midday, crave a nap in late afternoon, and feel fatigued in the evening. To reenergize, we grab a snack, but even when we watch what we eat—or maybe especially because we do—we're hungry an hour later and go back for more.

To meet our obligations and goals, we need to draw on substantial energy reserves so we can learn, remember, feel good, and perform well. Just as it is with our cars, it's the quality of the fuel we put in our tanks that determines how smoothly we run. And it's obvious from the way we so often feel exhausted, unable to concentrate, and out of gas (to continue the metaphor) that our diets don't provide us with what we need.

You'd think that selecting and consuming foods that make us feel refreshed and think clearly would be a snap to most of us. After all, it's been years since the USDA unveiled its Food Pyramid and bookshelves are full of best-selling diet plans that guarantee health and fitness to anyone buying into their advice. Of course, these programs often contradict each other and their lack of success is obvious to anyone who's scanned a newsstand, the Internet, or a crowd lately: About two-thirds of all adults are now overweight or obese, and roughly one in three kids and teens are or are close to being overweight.

The reason these plans haven't worked is because they don't make the connection between *feeding the brain* and *feeding the body*, and how the chemistry of the mind affects our physical needs. The problem isn't that we're not willing to work to improve our eating habits. The problem is that the diet plans themselves don't work, because they're not based on the most recent clinical research available from the scientific community about the mind-body connection and how the *chemistry of the brain* affects the *chemistry of the physique*.

Fortunately, the book you have in your hands is. *BrightFoods*, which cites nearly 900 medical journal sources, shows how foods, even those that are lumped in the same category, affect the brain and body differently. It demonstrates why other plans leave you hungry and vulnerable to scarfing down foods rich in empty calories, which make you feel listless, unsatisfied, and prone to over-eating. Designed by a neuropsychiatrist, it identifies the nutrient sources that not only provide high energy and the ability to focus, but leave you pleasantly satiated and able to get through the day without yielding to the siren call of hunger. By learning how food works with your body and mind, you can maintain them so they run with maximum efficiency and don't let you down.

The benefits of following the *BrightFoods* program are substantial. If you're an employee, it means being able to concentrate better at work, optimize your potential, and achieve more in the workplace. To employers, it means saving money lost to worker absenteeism due to lifestyle-related illnesses, which costs billions annually. Our kids should be able to feel healthier, miss fewer school days, and follow class-work better. And we can all expect to get more enjoyment out of our pastimes and passions, instead of slogging through the day absorbed in thoughts of snacks and sleep.

You don't have to be a scientist to appreciate *BrightFoods*. You just need a body and mind that you want to perform like a well-oiled machine. Consider this an owner's manual.

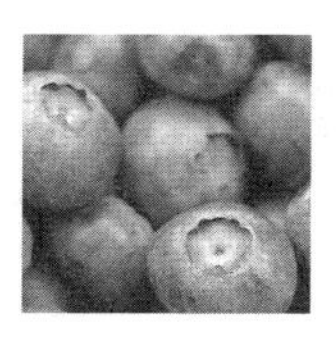

CHAPTER ONE
How Healthy Brain Cells Help Us Learn

When you eat, you're not just refueling your body: You're feeding your brain. Just as your body needs the right balance of nutrients to be healthy and grow, your brain requires the right combination of foods so it can perform optimally, too.

Luckily for us, the scientific community's understanding of this connection between quality nutrition and the brain's ability to work well has grown by leaps and bounds in recent years. Though it seems obvious to us now, it wasn't until 1672 that a physician named Thomas Willis first suggested that the brain was where our thoughts—the ability to imagine, remember, and experience sensations—took place, instead of, say, in the heart.

Today we might think of the brain as the computer hardware, and the mind (our thoughts) as its software; the software can be updated, but it can't run unless the hardware is in good working order. To appreciate why certain foods help us focus, learn, and perform far better than others, it helps to understand how that personal computer inside our heads operates.

The Mind Is a Learning Machine

If you took high school biology, you may have been taught that you were born with a limited number of fragile and irreplaceable brain cells, the building blocks containing enzymes that convert food to usable energy. Today, though, scientists know that the brain is made up of about 100 billion brain cells, each with about 10,000 synapses, or gaps between message transmitters and receivers, linking it to the others. These work together as a kind of computer "motherboard," only better, because brain cells can grow the more they're used.

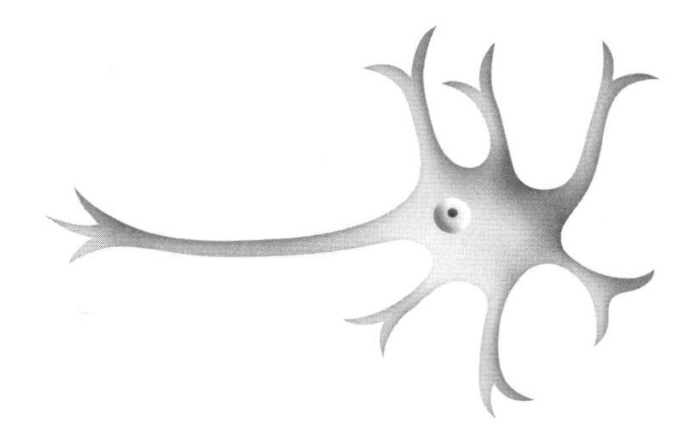

Just as your computer hard drive records information you type on your keyboard, your brain takes in data all the time. Our five senses constantly pass information along to our brains. Even when some don't function—for example, as was the case with the deaf and blind Helen Keller—information continues to be processed from the others (touch, taste, and smell) and stored as memories.

Then, when you think of a word such as "diving," your mind conducts a search and "sees," "hears," "smells," "tastes," and "touches" the experience of diving, or "views" documentary clips of the experience. Divers who've seen a whale shark might remember that image and "re-feel" the powerful emotions that have been in storage for years. This makes it possible to express the recalled information and emotions through art, music, speech, and writing.

Just as Helen Keller relied on her sense of touch, which sent information from her skin to her brain, it's possible to improve the way you get information through a particular sense when you focus, concentrate, and go slowly. Taking the time to read a document carefully instead of scanning it haphazardly increases the chances that you'll recall its contents a week later. If you clear your mind and practice tuning out distractions, as skilled physicians do to detect illness based on sounds in the abdomen, chest, and neck, you'll strengthen your listening skills. Food critics cultivate a heightened sense of taste; firemen learn to detect dangerous fumes and gases through reliance on their sense of smell.

Through our senses and repeated exposure to different types of stimulation, we often form impressions about the world around us without even realizing it. When we hear thunder outside, we learn to associate the sound with the lightning, clouds, darkness, and rain that we see. When a child observes that her mother is more likely to indulge her when she's in a good mood, she'll wait for the right moment before asking for a second dessert. A preschooler who became afraid of swings after falling off one will give it another try after seeing and hearing his buddies swing gleefully and without fear.

Other times, learning is a conscious process that requires concentration and effort. Some people prefer to gather information through reading. When they buy furniture and "some assembly" is required, they read the directions through before diving in. Others would rather learn by doing, and take a stab at putting the chest together on their own, knowing that they might have to start all over again. This isn't the wrong way to go, only a different way. After all, major discoveries such as Teflon have been made by people who didn't follow directions.

Twenty-four hours a day, the marvelous machinery of our brain works to help us navigate our lives. It takes in information gathered from the five senses and sorts it, assesses its importance and stores it for future use. It helps us concentrate on the task at hand—scanning a crowd to find a relative, pouring volatile chemicals—while filing away impressions we weren't even aware we were making at the time (whether it was hot or cold out, the people standing next to us). If our mission is interrupted by a fire alarm, the flexible brain is able to switch gears and recall what we've learned about fire alarms in the past, react to the situation, and then file away any new information we picked up before leaving the building.

The Mood-Learning Connection

Scientists who have examined the effects of different emotions on learning believe that when we feel serene and content, we're more likely to retain information and perform better. Research links positive outlooks to a part of the brain known as the left prefrontal cortex. In studies using brain scanners, monks who were highly skilled in meditation and led exceptionally positive and peaceful lives showed an increased amount of activity in this part of their brains.

Researchers have also linked negative emotions, such as worry, irritability, and anxiety, to the prefrontal cortex on the *right* side of the brain. In the same way that positive emotions seem to stimulate the left prefrontal cortex, experiencing negative feelings on a regular basis can increase activity in this area of the brain. Negative emotions behave like static on a television screen when it comes to learning, memory, and performance. They can interrupt the flow of incoming information and its processing.

We've all experienced the feelings that can muddle our abilities to focus and learn, one of the most common of which is depression, or unhappiness. When we're unhappy, we're likely to be tired and listless, due to under-activated brain cells. We take less interest in pleasurable activities, and may daydream or stare out the window or at the book we can't seem to finish, and we don't retain much of what we've covered. If we're fatigued or overwhelmed, our hearts may be into the goals we're trying to achieve, but we can't muster the energy to finish them. If we're sad because we feel inadequate and have low self-esteem, we may not see the point in focusing, think "what's the use" and give up.

On the other hand, if we're unhappy because we feel anxious, critical, pessimistic, judgmental, grouchy or worrisome, it's probably due to over-excited brain cells. All these negative emotions detract from our ability to feel good and learn. And there are significant health downsides: Over time, persistent anxiety can lead to fidgeting, headache, intestinal and chest discomfort, and neck and back tension; obsessive fretting leaves us emotionally exhausted and often sleepless.

Strengthening the Brain with a Good Workout

The more we use our memory, the stronger it becomes, and the larger it grows. For example, research indicates that people who memorized enormous amounts of information over a prolonged period of time showed an enlarged hippocampus, a part of the brain involved in learning and memorization, as measured by a brain scanner. It's now believed that this is due to brain circuit reorganization, increased brain cell connections or networking, and possibly the creation of new brain cells.

Until very recently, this was unthinkable. But we now understand that healthy brain cells can grow and flex like Silly Putty. We refer to this as "plasticity." The more we learn, the larger our memories become, in terms of both the amount of information stored and actual physical size.

And there's another way our brains can grow. The more we use our muscles, the more we add to the size of corresponding brain areas, and to a lesser extent, the entire brain. For example, avid violin players need enormous amounts of muscle strength in their left fingers to hold down thick cords. When they build up those muscles, the location of the brain cells controlling these strengthened fingers enlarges over time. In the same way, someone who constantly needs to use his right hand increases the size of the corresponding area of his brain. Athletes can not only increase the size of areas of the brain associated with their largest muscle groups, but also increase activity throughout the brain. As with memory, the more we use our bodies, the more our brains reorganize networks, and grow.

All the feats that the brain can achieve—learning through the senses, memorizing and storing information, feeling positive, and growing through steady use of our muscles—work best when we eat the optimal combinations of foods, and get the right amount of energy flowing through our well-maintained brain circuits. There's a name for this scientifically-designed, best of all possible eating plans: *BrightFoods.*

Chapter Summary

- It wasn't until 1672 that the scientific community began to understand how our thought processes emanate from the brain.
- Learning relies on input from the senses, information processing in a positive mood, and storage in brain cell circuits.
- Rigorous memory, physical or spiritual exercises invigorate corresponding areas of the brain in particular, and to a lesser extent, the brain in general.
- The brain continuously changes its circuitry, expands its network and may even make new brain cells; this expansion potential is called "plasticity."

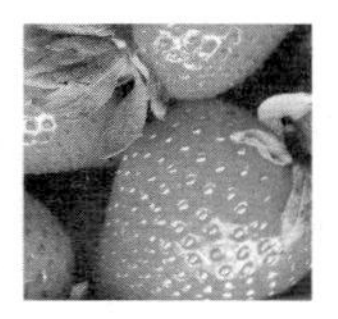

CHAPTER TWO

Brain Cells Work for *BrightFoods*: How Food Affects Learning, Memory, Mood, and Performance

All calories are not created equal, as anyone who's gobbled down a giant-sized muffin at 4 p.m., thinking that this snack will energize them for the next few hours, knows. At first you feel pleasantly full, but in no time, it's hard to concentrate, and you feel an overwhelming urge to take a nap. This is because foods affect thought in different ways. Some enhance brain cell plasticity and the ability to think, while others lead to brain cell corrosion and problems with learning, memory, mood, and performance.

Remember the lesson high school biology teachers used to pass on about the brain having a finite number of cells that broke on a daily basis and could not be replaced? It's true that some do get damaged, through head trauma, alcohol, drug use, oxygen deprivation, and even normal aging (though not nearly to the extent that was once thought). But now it's understood that brain cells don't really break, and that losing them doesn't lessen your intellectual abilities. Instead, each cell has a dimmer switch that is more under your control, through diet, exercise, and intellectual and spiritual stimulation, than previously suspected. So you don't experience breakage so much as you experience brown-outs!

How can you avoid brown-outs and keep the brain wattage bright, even into old age? We know that at about 60 percent fat, the brain is the fattiest organ in the body, and that all those billions of brain cells need a steady supply of oxygen and glucose—the blood sugar that's the main source of energy to the body—to transmit messages efficiently. When the glucose supply is disrupted, you experience brain cell brown-outs and have a harder time paying attention, you feel moodier, and you can't seem to get past your howling hunger pangs and food cravings.

To help you understand how this works, let's compare the energy requirements of your brain to that of your computer. Your computer's CPU (its energy source) hums along when fed a constant supply of 120 volts of electricity. When there's a power surge or dip in voltage, things can go haywire: the hard-drive can burn out and you can lose data. And the same thing happens to the brain cells in the mind. As long as they receive a steady infusion of oxygen, glucose, smart protein, and vital oils, they hum along, your mood stays even, and you're not aware of any cravings.

But when chemical balances get out of whack, things can go haywire in your brain, too. If the brain cells receive a power surge caused by an infusion of rapidly absorbed glucose—think of the giant muffin—you get a "sugar high." Alarms sound in the brain that sometimes overcorrect the problem, and a power dip results, because now the brain is running on too little glucose. The result: Just like your computer when there's a power surge, you crash. And if your diet doesn't include enough smart proteins or vital oils to help brain cells transmit, process, and store information, you're likely to feel distracted, fatigued, moody, and unlikely to learn or perform well. One thing will be on your mind, and that's satisfying your hunger.

What's in a Craving?

At *BrightFoods*, we believe that a craving is the brain screaming for an energy boost, or the desire to restore some missing vital nutrient so you can feel better. In *BrightFoods* language, hunger, cravings, and addictions are the same thing, because they're caused by the same lack of enough high-quality nutrients, and because they're resolved when you get a steady infusion of them.

In fact, food addictions can be *more powerful* than other kinds of addictions, and more difficult to conquer. Why? Although it's not easy, a cocaine addict or a cigarette- smoker can conquer his addictions by going cold turkey if he has enough nutritional, medical, and emotional support. People with poor eating habits, however, must continue to eat and at the same time literally relearn how to do it in a *BrightFoods*-friendly way.

The *BrightFoods* plan offers the kind of balanced nutritional, physical, and spiritual support that quiets the screams of those brain cells. Once they quiet down, the "user" is better able to concentrate, enjoy a more pleasant mood and meet her personal goals.

What Do Brain Cells Snack On? *BrightFoods* Nutrition and the Brain

BrightFoods recommends an array of foods that optimize the brain's ability to send and receive messages, reorganize, network, and stay plastic, thereby avoiding the brown-outs that cause hunger, cravings, and decreased focus and performance. In addition to a steady moderate flow of glucose provided by slowly-absorbed carbohydrates and sugars, such as those found in 100 percent stone ground wheat, brain cells love to snack on the following nutrients:

Smart Proteins

Brain cells enjoy light protein snacks found in minimally processed grains, vegetables, beans, poultry, lean meats, nuts, and eggs. Smart protein is converted into substances that are essential to thought, called amino acids; some of these become neurotransmitters, or cell-to-cell information messengers, which prepare brain cells to receive information.

There are scores of different types of information messengers, each functioning like a particular psychiatric "medicine" floating around in the brain. Some, including dopamine, norepinephrine, serotonin, the endorphins, and acetylcholine, may be familiar. Dopamine, a protein derivative, affects brain cell plasticity, improves focus, and can make you feel anywhere from pleasant to thrilled. Dopamine and norepinephrine come from the amino acid and smart protein tyrosine, which is found in meat, minimally-processed grains, beans, produce, and other foods. Serotonin, another information messenger, serves as a kind of "natural" antidepressant, sleeping pill, and anti-anxiety agent. It's found in turkey meat, certain produce, and warm milk in the form of tryptophan, a smart protein link that changes into serotonin. Tryptophan is the main reason why overeaters wind up on the couch after Thanksgiving dinner. Endorphins, generated by vigorous exercise and certain foods, are like the brain's heroin, and are responsible for "runner's high" or "athlete's zone," but they also increase your appetite. Not all messengers are made directly from amino acids, however. Acetylcholine, which enhances memory, is an important messenger that comes from egg yolks.

These nutrients, when eaten in moderation, make more messengers available, which speeds up communications on the brain-wide web. When brain cell communication is humming, so are you. You're calm and focused, and your mood is stable, meaning you experience fewer power dips and surges, cravings and feelings of unmanageability or hunger. But smart proteins don't do the job alone.

Vital Oils

While many oils and all saturated fats corrode the brain's hardware and compromise your ability to think, brain cells do love to "nibble" on a small and balanced buffet of vital oils. But they don't want large amounts of one vital oil straight-up, or from just any source. They function best when the vital oils arrive together in minimally-processed forms, such as filtered extra virgin olive oil, which we'll refer to as "olive oil"; a little of this stuff goes a long way. Certain other food sources, such as fatty fish and pressed flaxseed oil, are said to contain vital oil, but olive oil, greens, avocadoes, and walnuts may do a better job of delivering the kind of performance that keeps brain cells happy and humming. When eaten in combination with other foods, vital oils not only maintain, but can also significantly upgrade your memory and your brain's flexibility.

Antioxidants

Often, we eat certain foods that aren't optimal for good brain function. These foods leave behind a lot of harmful waste called free radicals that can damage many organs in the body, including brain cells. In fact, free radical damage can result in brain cell "rust," brown-outs, aging, and even brain cell death. To counteract this, we need antioxidants, which neutralize the free radicals and destroy them before they can take their "corrosive" action. The *BrightFoods* plan is high in antioxidant-rich foods that are minimally-processed, and pack a punch inside the body. These are usually more effective than antioxidant-containing foods that have been heavily processed, such as enriched flour, which may not have the power to vaporize the free radicals that emerge.

When you avoid blackening, frying, and dark-browning while cooking these foods, you do even more to upgrade your brain's hardware and software yet another notch.

Addictive Drugs vs. Curative Medicines

Why are some foods habit-forming or "addictive," while others are "medicinal"? Most likely, for the same reason that some drugs are thought of as addictive, and others medicinal. Oxycodone, for example, relieves physical and emotional pain, but when it wears off, both miseries return, with interest. The resulting crisp, fresh, physical and emotional pain reflects brain cells screaming for mercy, and for more oxycodone.

Cocaine, which is equally addictive, stimulates brain cells in a different way—by bathing them in dopamine. This initially produces joy, heightened productivity, and a riveting focus that can last up to ten minutes. But after that, the brain cells go into a freefall of roller coaster-sized proportions, and the famous cocaine "crash" begins. Starved for dopamine, these exhausted and scorned brain cells produce signals that feel like suicidal depression, physical and emotional exhaustion, and disorganized thinking. All they want is more, more, more!

Alcohol and marijuana work somewhat differently, by offering a sort of "virtual reality mini-vacation." Both substances are readily available and often used after a hard day's night or weekend victory, as a leisure activity, before, with or after food, or out of boredom. These addictive substances wrap users into a psychic space capsule and temporarily transport them far from what ails them. As a result, their performance levels will inevitably go way down, and they'll pay a big price the next day, when they can't think straight, their minds are sluggish, and they feel more irritable, impatient, intolerant, and anxious.

These withdrawal symptoms from alcohol and pot then become the perfect prompt for the next "very stressful" day. Make no mistake: Anyone who indulges in these flights from reality and then complains about his "stressful job" is misinterpreting what's going on. In such cases, we are not victims of stress; we choose to "do stress" as a down payment on the need for our next virtual mini-vacation.

Nicotine, when delivered via the most efficient drug-delivery system known to the body—smoking—works like a combination of Ritalin, Prozac, and a low dose of Valium, which are prescribed for attention deficit hyperactivity, depression, and muscle relaxation, respectively. The desired feeling lasts for about ten minutes. Then hundreds of thousands of brain cells scream out poignantly in a nicotine fit, calling for relief from attention deficit, fatigue, memory impairment, and increased body tension.

The reason these drugs are addictive is that they are used repeatedly over an extended period of time, until users begin to feel that ingesting them is the only reliable way to "feel better." At this point, use or abuse becomes dependence, because the ability to "choose" whether to use or not has been lost. Even though the individual is aware that the relief is temporary and whatever ails him will come back to haunt him, he feels compelled to continue this repetitive self-defeating behavior. Addicted people are *willing* to stop, but because addiction has robbed them of choice, they are *unable* to stop.

Curative Medicines

People take lots of medicines every day and don't become addicted to them. Millions who suffer from hypertension, for example, take medicines for high blood pressure, yet nobody has ever craved high blood pressure medicine. Diabetics take insulin or oral medicine every day, yet you never hear of anyone getting even the slightest urge for insulin or metformin. Depressives suffering from moderate to severe unhappiness take antidepressants, but no one craves these medicines either. The reason we don't become addicted to these curative medicines is simple: They help correct a deviation in the brain or body, and do nothing else. End of story.

Viewing Nutrients the *BrightFoods* Way

Addictive Foods

There are certain foods that cause changes in brain cell function resulting in desirable feelings, but then these good feelings give way to undesirable and uncomfortable emotions or withdrawal symptoms. When we eat too much of these foods, they clog up the messenger signals from one brain cell to another by making reorganization, networking, and plasticity more difficult, and lead to a lack of focus, drive, contentment, and easiness, and to increased cravings. *BrightFoods* considers these foods addictive:

- Pulverized, over-processed grains such as "enriched flour" used to make white, "whole wheat," rye, and many other baked goods and snacks. Also, over-processed and refined foods such as instant mashed potatoes, oatmeal, and rice, and most cold breakfast cereals. (There are plenty of *Bright* alternatives to choose from.) The excess refining process strips grain of its nutritious and fibrous outer husks, and grinds naked grain to the consistency of confectioners' sugar. Processors essentially pre-cook potatoes, oatmeal, and rice—foods that are easy to digest—so the body absorbs them as glucose faster than it does granular sugar.

The resulting short-lived, feel-good glucose high mimics cocaine, because it's rapidly replaced by the well-known sluggish, inattentive, wilted, and up-tight glucose crash that leaves brain cells screaming an hour later, when they're hungry again, for another ride on the sugar-high roller coaster.

- Saturated fats. Instead of mimicking cocaine, saturated fats imitate alcohol. They can be soothing and calming, but they freeze brain cell plasticity. And like a car forced to run on the wrong fuel, these fats don't burn cleanly, and can leave us with a bit of a hangover as our brain cells moan; this may be because we're eating saturated fats and denying our bodies vital oils. The typical American brain has a surplus of addictive saturated fat and a marked deficiency in vital oils. This shortage makes it harder for brain cells to reorganize and network, leading to memory loss, unhappiness, impatience, hostility, impaired concentration, and attention deficit symptoms. It also compels us to make repeated "cheeseburger with fries"-type choices. But don't worry; bread and beef are on the *BrightFoods* menu.
- Excess salt can be an addictive food additive, because it affects brain cell messaging. And for every molecule of it that we eat, we gulp down two molecules of water. As many can testify, water retention contributes to bloating, and bloating leads to moodiness in both sexes, and cramps in women.

Why? It's not just our feet, hands, and bellies that swell. Consider the ramifications of a bloated brain, with the resulting changes in brain chemistry and no place to expand, since it's constrained by the hard bony skull. Perhaps that's why excess salt can often lead to irritability, tension, and anxiety in many people. Too much salt also has built-in "progression" and "feeding frenzy" characteristics—that is, we keep eating even though we're full, perhaps because salt excites taste buds and brain cells (more on this later), and makes "self-control" something to which we're just paying lip service (pun intended).

In other words, salt contributes to the way chips and fries fly down our esophagus like runaway trains, in contrast to their "no salt added" relatives. The ensuing salt-induced discomfort drives us to the next item on our binge list, as we search for relief.

- Sugar substitutes can leave the brain down and out of glucose. Low brain glucose means low energy and continued hunger. Although sugar substitutes have been cleared of potential cancer-forming properties, the havoc these chemicals may play with emotions, energy, ambition, and brain cell functioning has not been researched. Studies are lacking that show their usefulness in weight loss and maintenance or diabetes management. Some people, however, report weight gain as a by-product of using sugar substitutes, because like marijuana that's used without food, it doesn't satisfy hunger or cravings for glucose, protein or vital oils. So while you're saving calories, your appetite for a couple of slices of pizza and a meatball Parmegian submarine sandwich is intensifying. Smaller portions of our *Bright* pizza and sub equivalents are designed to be more satisfying.

It's cruel to satisfy the tongue but not the brain cells. Artificial sweeteners do just that: They may temporarily quench your psychological sugar craving, but do nothing for your biological energy needs. *BrightFoods* offers non-fattening alternatives to sugar substitutes for coffee and tea.

- Monosodium glutamate (MSG) is another food additive that shoots unfriendly missiles at brain cells and can impair their reorganization and networking, as well as the ability to think. When taken in excess, the compound can excite brain cells—that is, raise them to a higher energy level-to the point of death. Additives that can do this, including a derivative of the sugar substitute aspartame, are called "excitotoxins." Excess glutamate can not only excite the taste buds and lead to loss of self-control, just as salt does, but it also can stimulate the central nervous system and trigger feeding frenzies. In the *BrightFoods* dictionary, we define "feeding frenzy" as: "n. See cheese-coated chips and snacks."

Anyone who has ever suffered a headache or irritability from MSG infusion knows how weirdly uncomfortable that feeling can be, but most people don't make the connection between the additive and feeling lousy. Excess glutamate, and possibly aspartate, have been linked in some people to anxiety, panic, irritability, obsessive worry, unhappiness, inappropriate displays of anger and violence, and irritable bowel syndrome. Excess glutamate is liberally added to many processed convenience foods. It can also be formed naturally, when certain foods such as cheese or soy are heated or otherwise processed.

Viewed the *BrightFoods* way, it's no wonder these foods have the potential to provide emotional bliss, which is quickly followed by emotional turmoil and difficulty in learning and performing, as masses of besieged brain cells call out for relief from the withdrawal symptoms these foods create. When experiencing them, nothing spells relief better than M-O-R-E O-F T-H-E S-A-M-E.

Medicinal Foods

Medicinal foods, on the other hand, can fortify brain cell reorganization and networking, and also improve the mind's ability to think, be attentive, and feel energetic, while at the same time allowing you to perform at your best. How? Medicinal, slowly absorbed sugars deliver energy, attentiveness, mood stability, and drive in a steady and sustained way that leaves your brain cells quite content, with no hunger or urges for hours. Ask yourself: Have you ever heard of anyone dashing under the cover of darkness to an all-night convenience store to purchase bananas, uncooked fettuccine or old-fashioned oats?

Similarly, have you ever been at a party and tried eating an olive or two, then moving on to another activity? Compare that to trying to eat a potato chip or two and then focusing on anything else. Both are salty snacks loaded with fat, yet you can feel satisfied with a small amount of the first, and crave an enormous portion of the second. The kind of calories from fat that each contains either satisfies us or stimulates us with cravings for more.

Medicinal oils such as olive oil contain minimally-processed vital oils and antioxidants that burn cleaner in our bodies, reliably deliver a variety of fatty acids in healthier proportions, and become part of our brain cells, not our bellies. Like slowly- absorbed sugars, vital oils help stabilize mood, improve focus, endurance, memory, and ambition, can curb your appetite for saturated fats, and lead to improved performance. The vital oils mentioned above, which are linked to improved plasticity, combine with a steady supply of slowly-absorbed glucose, smart proteins, and oxygen to deliver exactly what your brain synapses need to communicate efficiently.

In the *BrightFoods* regimen, antioxidants work with other medicinal foods to reduce cravings by keeping brain cell corrosion to a minimum. Far from being a lot of health-food propaganda, the need for antioxidants is real, and *BrightFoods* explains where to get the ones researchers believe are still strong by the time they get inside your body.

We also recommend medicinal additives. Just as reducing your salt intake helps keep your mood stable, so does adding flavor-enhancing, fresh or dried 100 percent natural herbs and spices such as pepper, mustard, and turmeric.

Overall, *BrightFoods* recommends a balance of various medicinal foods to optimize the brain's ability to send and receive messages, and to avoid the brown-outs that cause cravings and problems with thinking. When given the right nutritional support, the brain can reignite nerve cell connections that have been clogged by sugar swings, excess or poor protein intake, saturated fat, and ruinous free radicals. The plastic brain can create new or restored pathways that can reduce cravings, restore vitality, and aid children and adults who have occasional inattentiveness, or chronic attention deficit hyperactivity disorder, to focus. The *BrightFoods* plan can also improve concentration in forgetful people, as well as those suffering from full-blown dementia.

It's likely that, in the future, science will discover even more instances in which solid nutrition can benefit growth—perhaps in the service of transforming stem cells inside our brain into new brain cells. Stay tuned.

Dieting: A Theory

As we've stated, once you crave addictive foods, you lose the ability to choose medicinal foods over addictive foods, causing shortages of slowly-absorbed glucose, smart proteins, antioxidants, and vital oils. It's for this reason, we believe, that diet pills haven't been effective in helping users achieve ideal weight and keep the pounds off over time. In addition, most diet pills have mood-altering side effects that intensify already-existing food cravings. Most importantly, the diet pills of tomorrow are doomed to follow the present diet pill path, unless someone figures out how they can deliver minimally-processed, slowly-absorbed glucose, smart proteins, vital oils, and antioxidants in small amounts during waking hours.

After all, we all want the same thing: a mind that can focus well and solve problems, housed in a calm and relaxed body. When you choose medicinal foods, you're free to decide when you want and what you want to eat, because you're not driven by hunger and out-of-control cravings. Instead of choosing addictive foods that perpetually make you feel disappointed and guilty, your food selections become much more voluntary and satisfying.

Extra! Food Pyramid Collapses

A decade or so ago, our government responded to statistics from the Centers for Disease Control indicating that heart disease, overweight and obesity are the chief killers of our fellow Americans. After consulting with a vast number of experts, health officials advised us to eat a low-fat diet.

The country swung into action, nutritionally speaking. The United States Department of Agriculture revised the Food Pyramid to include lots of starches and very little fat, and made no distinction between good fats and bad fats, or complex carbohydrates and slowly-absorbed glucose. Misguided food manufacturers took the recipes of our favorite foods and produced low-fat versions, replacing the fat with more fat-producing and heart-taxing rapidly-absorbed carbohydrates. Convenience food-makers made low-fat food tasty by adding heapings of salt and using ingredients that are not only unpronounceable, but are also not found in nature.

We consumers played our part by putting our lives into the hands of government agencies who were trying to appease both politicians, some with conflicting interests, and consumers. Meanwhile, most of the food processors didn't have a conscientious medical nutritionist on staff to advise them.

America has much strength, but when it comes to inventing a healthier way of eating, we're definitely not the sharpest tool in the worldwide shed. The very convenience-oriented technologies and industries that have made us the envy of the world have also made us the most overweight and obese, in terms of the percentage of population affected. The myriad emotional and medical diseases associated with obesity are choking us financially, not to mention the fact that many of us will eventually be killed by them. As citizens of other countries gradually adopt our way of eating, immigrants to these shores are beginning to show higher incidences of disease, too.

The Food Pyramid's architects meant well. Nevertheless, we now know that if we adhere to it, with its glut of over-processed foods, addictive carbohydrates, and lack of vital oils, antioxidant foods and additives, smart proteins, and slowly absorbed carbohydrates, our brains are on a straight path to becoming "plaster." We're also more susceptible to disorganized thinking, mood swings, sluggishness, anxiety, worry, craving, obesity, and a whole host of medical illnesses, including premature death.

Trying to live a healthful life via the Food Pyramid, even as it was reconfigured in January 2005, practically guarantees one thing: long-term nutritional failure. The *BrightFoods* way of life, in contrast, enhances thinking and health, and is a lifelong pleasure, not the flavor of the month.

In the end, it really doesn't matter whether cancer, heart disease, or obesity is listed as the number one cause of death. It is, however, vital to realize that addictive disorders involving eating, smoking, and drinking can lead to brain dysfunction, obesity, cancer, and heart disease.

Why Most Eating Plans Eventually Lead You to the Next One

You can put away your calculator, because counting calories is not part of the *BrightFoods* plan. We have been brainwashed into thinking that "low calorie" equals better health and weight loss, and that "high calorie" equals weight gain and disease. It's time to take another look.

Once you think the *BrightFoods* way, you see the counting-calorie fallacy. A simple example: One sugar packet, 56 grams, has 210 calories. One hundred and twelve grams of fettuccine has 400 calories. Most of us believe that 210 calories of granular sugar is less fattening than 400 calories of fettuccine, when in fact the reverse may be true. Granular sugar is absorbed and burns rapidly like a dish of kerosene, and al dente cooked fettuccine absorbs slowly and burns like an oak log. Which one would you rather have to warm your Wyoming lodge in February? Because table sugar is rapidly absorbed and more readily causes a glucose spike requiring insulin to store the excess spillage, a large percentage of those unburned granular sugar calories is converted into fat. The fettuccine, on the other hand, becomes sustained, energizing brain fuel that burns more slowly, produces no sugar spikes or excess spillage, and therefore causes much less or essentially no conversion to fat—even at almost double the number of calories and grams consumed.

Eating addictive "low calorie" products leaves you looking for more, and hungry within an hour. Eating medicinal foods doesn't. That's why calories are essentially meaningless as long as they are medicinal calories. The same holds true for energy-producing, appetite-suppressing olive oil.

Another reason low calorie diets don't work is because they can contribute to malnutrition, which can make your concentration, mood, and energy low, while at the same time increasing anxiety, irritability, hunger, bingeing, and weight. *BrightFoods* eating changes all that.

Simply stated, low-carbohydrate, low-calorie, low-fat diets haven't proven to be effective in helping most of us reach and maintain ideal weight. Maybe it's because these diets tend to leave us with lower levels of essential nutrients, and increase hunger, cravings for rapidly-absorbed carbohydrates and saturated fat, and over-eating. These diets make carbohydrates, calories, protein, and fat our focal points. They don't take into account vital oil ratios, how rapidly some sugars and carbohydrates become glucose, where the protein comes from, antioxidant deficiencies, and hidden, unpronounceable additives that can breed learning and behavioral trouble.

On the other hand, diets that emphasize eating a lot of protein and fat don't work either, because they choke the brain cells of the glucose they need, don't deliver enough vital oils, and dim the wattage. When eaten over long periods of time, menus that are heavy in saturated fats, and often high in additives and low in antioxidants, hurt brain cells, and leave the brain exposed to unchecked free-radical bombardment. Just like the diet that's heavy in rapidly absorbed carbohydrates, this kind of eating also breeds thinking and behavioral problems, and makes you feel dissatisfied and yearning to binge on carbohydrates.

Probably the main reason we persist in counting calories is the popular belief, adopted by the new Food Pyramid and exercise recommendations, that obesity and overweight are due to an imbalance between caloric intake and physical activity. But that assumption can be viewed another way: The more low-calorie, highly-processed, and additive-rich foods we consume, the more we feel fatigued, bored and anxious, lack drive and want to procrastinate. This state of mind makes physical activity close to impossible, and the recommendation to increase physical activity under these circumstances is easier said than done. In addition, exercising while obese can be hazardous to your health, as we'll discuss in a later chapter. Exercise might be most beneficial after the obese person has lost a lot of weight, and his physician has signed off on his workout plan.

What Does *BrightFoods* Deliver?

Because *BrightFoods* teaches you to use food to quiet your distracting cravings, it can release you from years of self-defeating and guilt-ridden inner struggle. It's okay to eat when you feel hungry. When you eat more foods that are medicinal and nonhabit-forming every few hours, you supply the brain with reliable high-quality nutrients that help you focus, process information, and set priorities, and you won't feel the need to plan for your next hunger attack. You're more likely to accomplish scheduled tasks, solve problems quickly and efficiently, and feel satisfied all day long.

Because *BrightFoods* recommends reducing the amount of addictive additives you take in, you'll have less damaging brain toxicity and feel more clear-headed and calmer. Most likely, you'll also become more patient and accepting, and less likely to feel impulsive, argumentative, and resentful.

Because *BrightFoods* is high in antioxidants that are believed to work inside your body, thereby helping brain cell reorganization and networking, the plan can have anti-aging benefits as well, and keep you happy, bright, and functioning well your entire life. And because *BrightFoods* can give you more energy, you can experience a greater sense of accomplishment, think more creatively and inventively, and become more involved in family life, work, and leisure activities. Because *BrightFoods* can leave you feeling happier, you may find yourself grateful for what you have, instead of focusing on what you don't have. You're likely to be less critical and more accepting of others, more socially interactive, and have better relationships with family members, friends, peers, and clients.

Because *BrightFoods* helps you feel your best, arrive at the weight you want and keep you there, you can lower your risk of developing many forms of cancer, cardiovascular disease, hypertension, stroke, diabetes, Alzheimer's disease, and premature death.

How can you resist getting into *BrightFoods*?

Chapter Summary

- Brain cells don't die off as much as they undergo brown-outs.
- Brown-outs are associated with poor thinking and decreased performance.
- *BrightFoods* divides foods and additives into two basic categories: addictive and medicinal.
- Medicinal foods pamper brain hardware and plasticity, and are mind-friendly, improving learning, memory, mood, and performance.
- Feeling hungry or having cravings is the way your brain screams for an energy boost, or for correcting your balance of nutrients when you're on a diet rich in addictive ingredients.
- The best way to avoid brown-outs and the inattentiveness, moodiness, fatigue, and hunger they can cause is by feeding brain cells small amounts of medicinal foods every few hours.
- A *Bright* meal or snack enjoyed every few hours throughout the day boosts energy and prevents nutrient shortages, thereby keeping hunger and cravings at bay while enhancing learning, memory, mood, and performance.

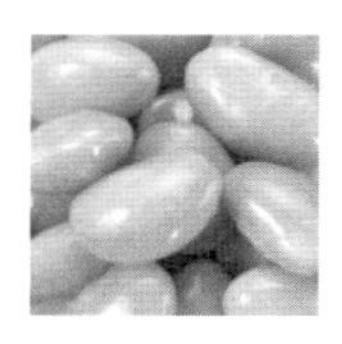

CHAPTER THREE
Brighten Your Mind: Reduce Brain Rust

"Leave your drugs in the chemist's pot if you can heal the patient with food."
—HIPPOCRATES

You've probably heard a lot of talk, and a lot of confusion, about the importance of antioxidants—substances such as Vitamin C and lycopene that protect body cells from the damage caused by excited oxygen molecules. And it's no wonder, since healthcare providers constantly urge us to "eat more fruits, vegetables, and whole grains," and imply that these foods—processed or otherwise-all contain the same health-sustaining properties.

So we turn to fad diet books for information, and consume food products and supplements we're told are good for us. But the authors, manufacturers, and vendors we rely on are often misleading about which foods are best.

The truth is, not all foods and supplements that contain antioxidants outside the body retain their medicinal potency once they're ingested. Similarly, unprocessed foods can lose their antioxidant properties through processing. It's important to make this distinction, because it's the antioxidant-containing foods that work best in the body that play a key role in keeping you healthy. The ones we recommend have been selected based on medical research, and form one of the four essential *BrightFoods* groups. They slow down the aging process, improve focus, learning, memory, mood, and performance, and clean up the brain rust that can impede clear thinking.

What Is Brain Rust?

"Brain rust" is a term we use to describe the toll that excited oxygen molecules take on brain cells. Where do these unwanted oxygen molecules come from? They're called free radicals, and they're mainly by-products of burning the thousands of food calories—human fuel—that we use each day to keep trucking along. Just like cars, we need fuel to function properly. The mind never stops burning fuel, even while we're resting, meditating or sleeping. And just as it is when we drive, whenever we burn through our energy sources, we create a corresponding amount of emissions in the form of free radicals, causing brain rust—or, as it's referred to in the scientific community, "oxidative stress," or "cell aging."

We all have brain rust. This corrosion occurs in every cell of the brain, starts forming even before we're born and continues each day throughout our lives. But when too much accumulates, our minds can't work at full capacity, and we're more susceptible to disease. We need to eat foods that help eliminate the free radicals that cause brain rust.

Some medical nutritionists argue that consuming fewer calories leads to less free radical formation. But not having enough energy to run on is a big price to pay for decreased emissions, especially since there are ways to help neutralize free radical pollutants in our brains and still have the energy we need to achieve our goals.

Another strategy—limiting our gassing up to three times a day and possibly over-filling it during those times—doesn't necessarily make the brain run more efficiently, either. Our meals and snacks need to contain enough calories from the *right combination* of foods—balanced amounts of antioxidants, vital oils, smart proteins, and slowly-absorbed glucose (more on these last three in future chapters). If the food we eat is high in saturated fats, animal protein, and toxic additives, our brains rust and conk out. Just like it sounds, this makes it difficult to stay on task, learn, remember, perform, and maintain a good mood.

That's why the *BrightFoods* way to fuel up our brains is to eat a little at a time, 16/7. We believe it is the healthiest method for keeping energy steadily flowing through well-maintained brain cell circuits all day and through the evening, for the rest of our lives. This eating pattern results in the lowest amount of free radical formation, and the highest fuel efficiency and best mind performance possible.

How Free Radicals Work and How We Defeat Them

To understand why the *BrightFoods* plan succeeds in minimizing destructive free radicals where other programs fail, you need to understand how they work. So here's a brief organic chemistry lesson to help you appreciate how the program improves your health and brain function (we promise to keep it short and sweet).

Free radicals are oxygen molecules with unpaired electrons, which make them excited and more unstable than molecules in which the electrons all have partners. Electrically unstable oxygen molecules are harmful to cells and DNA, and can even lead to cancer formation. We can think of them as machine gun-toting terrorists who take pot shots at different parts of our brain cells, and damage them. And they don't stop there: They essentially target all living cells and organ systems in the body, leaving poor functioning, aging, and disease in their wake. About 10,000 times per day, one researcher estimates, countless legions of these terrorists attack the genetic information or DNA inside each cell throughout the body. When our bodies have accumulated too many free radicals, we refer to this as oxidative stress.

This can lead to multiple health problems. If free radicals aim at cholesterol, heart disease can develop. Having too many free radicals has also been associated with diabetes and its complications, skin cell damage and eventual skin cancer. If they target genetic material in the organ systems, they've been known to detonate cancer in them, too.

Although free radicals are everywhere, and no organ system can avoid their wrath, they prefer attacking the brain, because it's the fattiest organ in the body, and uses vast amounts of oxygen and glucose around the clock. This makes it the largest free radical factory and oxidative stress hot-bed in the body, since free radicals are formed where saturated fat, oxygen, and glucose interact.

The most common origin of free radicals, and their resulting brain rust, is our failure to completely burn up all the calories we take in, especially when they come from diets high in saturated fats, animal protein, and processed sugars, as these fuels don't burn clean. People who eat smaller, healthier meals and snacks more often are more likely to be clear-headed and feel better than people who consume low-calorie, low-carbohydrate or low-fat diets, or high-calorie Atkins-type meals. These can release legions of free radicals that pummel the mind and leave us feeling moody and bewildered.

The choice in the past has been between eating low-calorie meals and snacks that can leave us with a cleaner brain but hungry, with little fuel to get to where we're going, or to feel fuller by consuming a lot more calories, but at the same time producing more free radicals. But now there's a third, better choice. Each medicinal ingredient in *BrightFoods* meals and snacks has been selected and recommended in portions designed to keep free radical formation low and still leave us feeling satisfied, attentive, and energetic.

Calorie overload is a major cause of free radical formation, but there are others, such as cigarette-smoking. Another source that we can control is the way we cook our food.

Cooking Methods and Other Free Radical Sources

Although one of the major sources of free radicals is the calories we eat, other sources abound. Brain rust can result from baking, broiling, barbecuing or frying meats, fish, dairy products, and vegetables, because browned or burnt meats, oils, grains, and vegetables such as fries or chips increase toxins that lead to free radical formation. This happens when high temperatures break up electron pairs and generate more excited oxygen molecules, or free radicals. These cell-rusting substances add to overall brain and body oxidative stress, which has been linked to poor thinking and numerous types of cancers, including cancer of the breast, prostate, and colon.

The good news is that *BrightFoods* was designed by someone who's a meat lover and vegan (about a third of the year due to religious practices), not a soy and sprout-chomping extremist, so there's no need to sell the grill, or miss out on fried calamari or barbequed ribs. In fact, it's not necessary to stop eating your favorite addictive, free radical-forming foods completely, because you kill bacteria and may be keeping your body in tip-top shape by having some free radicals in you to challenge your immune system. These foods can be eaten from time to time, as long as you first ingest large amounts of antioxidant foods and 1000 mgs of vitamin C, or Ester-C if you have a sensitive stomach.

And if you're a steak-lover, you can enjoy your favorite food served up medium-rare to rare, because this way it contains less rust-forming properties. If you order it the extra-rusting well-done way, you can serve it up with counter-rust sides such as uncooked baby carrots and *BrightFoods* Smashed Potatoes (recipe found in Chapter Nine). It's best to avoid eating the fried or burnt parts of any type of food, but if it's unavoidable, you can counter its effects to some extent by taking in extra antioxidants and 1000 mgs of vitamin C.

Other foods you want to avoid include processed oil and soy; health and fitness foods; hormone and antibiotic residue in meats (free range or organic meats are options); food additives; mercury and dioxin in fish and fish supplements and pesticide residue in produce and supplements. (More on this later). Free radical-forming pollutants and toxins are also constantly entering the body through the air we breathe and the water we drink.

But have no fear. Trying to avoid free radical sources doesn't mean we have to give up our favorite foods or stop enjoying life. *BrightFoods* has identified a way to counter the toxic effects of addictive free radical-forming foods: by increasing portions of medicinal foods that improve our attentiveness and keep our academic ambitions high.

Free Radical Terminators to the Rescue

As we now know, antioxidants help clean up rust inside the brain and help us think better by reducing oxidative stress over time. They increase the brain cell's ability to grow and network, and boost the mind's capacity to focus, learn, memorize, and perform higher-order tasks, such as planning. They do this so well, in fact, that doctors have prescribed them as a medical treatment when a patient's ability to think is mildly diminished, as well as for those who have been severely impaired by Alzheimer's and other degenerative brain diseases.

If free radical terrorists carry machine guns, what do free radical terminators use to retaliate? They use "electron-lasers" to shoot electrically charged particles at free radicals, thereby changing unpaired electrons in excited oxygen molecules back into calm and stable couples. This is how antioxidants in foods neutralize the free radicals' ability to promote brain rust: When a free radical terminator is low on electron-laser ammo, she "borrows" from a buddy. We win the war that rages in our bodies between free radical terminators and brain cell terrorists when we consume a variety of antioxidants every day. Each day that we meet our quota of five servings of produce per day, derived mainly from whole foods, we win another battle on behalf of our brain's hardware and software, meaning there's more cell networking and growth going on.

It's a simple equation: When the number of newly-introduced free radical terminators (which we get mainly from whole foods) out-number the newly-formed free radical terrorists, the mind becomes brighter and quicker. That spells more efficient learning and recall, and better performance. You just need to eat more antioxidant-containing medicinal foods at each meal and snack than free radical-forming addictive foods. For example, eating a large salad with *BrightFoods* salad dressing and 500 mgs of vitamin C before eating a lean burger helps terminators triumph over free radicals.

Perhaps you could say I'm from Missouri, because *BrightFoods* touts a "show me" attitude when it comes to selecting antioxidants for our ingredient list. We do not blindly follow celebrities or "eat right" gurus. We check medical references before giving an antioxidant the *BrightFoods* seal of approval, because there is little doubt that antioxidants differ in free radical-terminating strength. Some are just imposters, and the same antioxidant—for example, Vitamin C in a fresh orange, a previously heated carton of orange juice, or various brands of vitamin C supplements—is absorbed by the body in different ways.

When we use the term "antioxidant" in this book, we're only referring to foods or supplements that can infiltrate the body and effectively help polish off those free radical beasties, because it doesn't matter how strong an antioxidant is *before* processing or entering the body. The potential of an antioxidant to absorb and exert its medicinal effect inside the human body is referred to as its "bioavailability."

It Isn't in, Until It's in

Some antioxidants can infiltrate free radical bunkers in both fresh and processed forms, as is the case with crushed garlic and processed garlic supplements. Others absorb better when accompanied by buddies such as vitamins C and E paired up with aloes. Research methods vary, so there are questions about the disease-fighting value of some organically grown foods compared with conventional produce, or those grown differently in other parts of the world. It's hard to evaluate study results when the antioxidant being tested comes from a variety of sources (think of our vitamin C example).

However they're ingested, though, a fresh, cooked, processed or encapsulated antioxidant can't do its work until it treks across the intestinal wall. But before we compare how five foods containing antioxidants perform in the body, let's look at a startling true story illustrating how the mildest difference in pill-packing can alter the way your body absorbs a prescription medicine:

> *Karen, a young wife and mother of two, was prescribed the brand name drug Prozac, which gave her the focus and extra ambition she wanted to efficiently juggle her daily events and challenges. After about a year of consistent and marked improvement, she was convinced by her pharmacist that the generic was "the same, only cheaper." A mere two days after switching to the generic form of Prozac, Karen felt suicidal. Her psychiatrist called in another prescription for the brand name Prozac, and Karen's scary bout with suicidal thoughts, the first in her life, ended soon after.*

How is this possible when brand and generic Prozac both contain exactly the same active ingredient, fluoxetine? The answer is bioavailability. Since many people don't have problems absorbing medicine when they switch from the brand name to the generic, it's possible that Karen's problem was due to her particular genetic makeup. Most likely, she couldn't absorb the drug well once it was combined with some pill-packing or inactive ingredient that wasn't present in the brand name Prozac.

And unlike brand name medicines, generics, over-the-counter medications and supplements don't have to undergo testing for absorption and bioavailability before they're sold. In fact, the differences in bioavailability between brand and generic drugs have also been documented in medical journals for blood thinning, heart, and seizure medications, as well as many others.

So what about the processed supplements, and fresh and processed, organic and conventional produce? Are the antioxidants we think we're getting hitting home-runs for us? We can look to medical research for answers.

Blueberries Are Good but No Great Shakes

In vitro studies—tests done *outside* the body—do in fact crown blueberries as antioxidant kings. But scientists now have the capacity to test an antioxidant's abilities to spar with free radicals *inside* the body, so they can distinguish between the real free radical terminators and the wanna-bes. So how did the little blue-purple beauties, which are colored by antioxidants called anthocyanins, hold up when challenged? When compared in the body to an antioxidant considered to be weaker, the strength of blueberries became a horse of a different color; only about one-tenth of the anthocyanin was assimilated into the body. That means that blueberries lose their antioxidant punch once they're inside the body.

There is also evidence that heating and processing affects the bioavailability of the anthocyanins found also in black raspberries, plums, highly-processed supplements and red wine as well. And speaking of wine, drinking moderate amounts or more of red wine is said to lower antioxidant levels in our blood (though the healthful antioxidants in red wine can be quite beneficial when imbibed in modest amounts). This, taken along with the fact that alcohol is also a risk factor for cancer when men drink more than two glasses per day and women more than one, suggests that there can be too much of a good thing.

All in all, these facts take anthocyanin-rich foods such as blueberries, blackberries, and physician-approved amounts of red wine down a notch in the antioxidant hierarchy, though they're still *BrightFoods*.

Did you ever think blueberries could be this complicated? Wait till you hear about spinach.

Popeye Could Have Been Even Smarter

Spinach is one antioxidant-rich food that seems to be sensitive to the slightest amount of processing. Though a major player in the war on free radicals, it loses a lot of power once it's heated. When steamed, this big boy becomes 25 percent weaker in its fighting power against free radicals, and it seems likely that its strength decreases even more when it's boiled, processed, canned, or made into an extract or powder and mixed with pill-packing.

Spinach contains many different types of antioxidants, and besides its calories, it contains iron, an additional source of free radicals. But the overall antioxidant punch of fresh spinach is very high, and more than a match for the free radicals that come from iron and burning up spinach calories. Middle-aged spinach leaves seem to be higher in phenolics and flavinoid, two types of antioxidant, than baby or older leaves, though we recognize that this is certainly tough for the consumer to gauge. When was the last time you asked a spinach leaf its age?

All in all, fresh spinach is a great antioxidant, and middle-aged organic spinach is ideal, but not necessary. The higher antioxidant content of fresh spinach and other produce should not take precedence over safety. Also, check with your doctor before eating green leafy vegetables if a blood thinner has been prescribed for you, because they contain vitamin K, which can interfere with your medication.

Empty Waves of Grain

Unprocessed whole wheat grain contains phenolics and other antioxidants. But before we start separating the wheat from the chafe in terms of what's good for you, let's examine the different parts of an ear of wheat.

The outer part of the wheat kernel is the bran, which is usually ripped off during refined milling. It contains smart protein, niacin, riboflavin, magnesium, iron, and fiber—the kind of unprocessed fiber that helps fight overweight and cancer (supplement fiber has been shown to be ineffective). The "body" of the kernel is made up of smart protein, slowly absorbed glucose, minerals, B vitamins, and fiber. The smallest part is the germ, and it contains vital oils, smart protein, fiber, vitamin E, riboflavin, thiamine, iron, and minerals. These three parts make whole wheat grain one of nature's most nutrient-packed medicinal foods *before it's processed* and put in the bread, buns, cakes, cold breakfast cereals, cookies, muffins, pastas, pitas, pizza crust, rolls, snacks, and wraps we eat. The antioxidant, fiber, vital oil, smart protein, and slowly-absorbed glucose removal begins with certain milling procedures.

It's crucial that breads and baked goods be milled properly to ensure that they're nutrient-rich medicinal foods containing bioavailable antioxidants. The best antioxidant-containing and over-all nutrient-preserving baked goods come from *stone mills*, because they grind slowly and in a cooler environment. Cooler grinding methods don't heat antioxidants and other nutrients as much, and preserve the medicinal value of the whole grains.

On the other hand, we usually buy bread, baked goods, and manufactured foods containing wheat flour that have been milled in a different way: at high speeds, using cylinder or hammer mills that can generate temperatures up to 150 degrees F. This process can destroy enzymes and nutrients, cause oxidation and change antioxidants and vital oils so they permit brain-rusting. The end result of cylinder or hammer milling can be ransacked flour that's low in antioxidants and nutrition. The resulting starch dust is so deficient that processed thiamin, riboflavin, niacin, and iron must be added for "enrichment."

And as if that weren't enough, enriched flour is often bleached after that with chlorine dioxide or benzoyl peroxide. And chlorine dioxide behaves just like free radicals.

Other additives may include methyl bromide, nitrogen trichloride, and nitrogen peroxide. Here's a good general *BrightFoods* rule: If an ingredient is difficult to pronounce, eat antioxidant-containing foods along with it, or just say no.

Even manufacturers would agree that none of these chemicals have one germ of antioxidant or nutritional value. A search of the scientific literature shows no significant association between bread, pasta or breakfast cereals made from "enriched flour" and increased antioxidant activity inside the body. This should come as no surprise, and unfortunately, if enriched flour is not part of the solution to brain rust, cancer, heart disease, and obesity, it may be part of the problem. To sum it up in a wheat-bran shell: With phrases like "100 Percent Whole Wheat" and "Multigrain" added, most commercial breads, buns, cakes, cold breakfast cereals, cookies, muffins, pastas, pitas, pizza crusts, rolls, snacks, and wraps may give us the misimpression that we're getting a lot more "whole grain" than we actually are.

In reality, the first listed or main ingredient in these products is either bleached enriched flour or enriched flour, and hiding behind the "whole wheat flour" ingredient façade doesn't make it more healthful. "Whole wheat flour" is most often a blend of bleached enriched flour and unbleached whole wheat flour, while the preferred first ingredient should read "100 percent stone-ground whole wheat flour."

In my opinion, the use of "enriched flour" in the American diet is nothing short of a nutritional felony, especially when products made from enriched flour make up such a large portion of the base of the Food Pyramid. This weakness in its foundation may eventually contribute to its collapse. In contrast, the *BrightFoods* Pyramid (Appendix I) is built on antioxidant-containing produce, legumes, nuts, vital oils, and whole grains, including stone ground whole wheat flour, wild rice, and old fashioned oat meal.

Because cylinder- or hammer-milled flour is depleted of antioxidants and other nutrients, *BrightFoods* has developed its own ideal nutrient-rich formula for breads, baked goods, and original recipes that uses flour containing 100 percent stone ground organic whole wheat, among two other antioxidant-containing ingredients. Check it out in the recipe section of Chapter Nine.

Iced Tea Rules When Made Fresh

Although debates continue as to which is stronger, black and green tea are both powerful antioxidants outside the body. Researchers also find that the antioxidants in tea remain very strong inside the body when made fresh and taken warm, or poured over ice. Other studies of the way tea affects the body report only modest increases in the antioxidant power of fresh tea. Still others, using purified or processed forms of tea, tea extracts, and different testing methods, have found that tea has limited antioxidant potential. This means that fresh tea contains more antioxidant strength than instant tea mixes, and canned or bottled preparations.

Tea contains powerful polyphenolic antioxidants that are indeed absorbed to different degrees, and are powerful weapons against free radicals. *BrightFoods* considers black, green, red or white tea to be bioavailable antioxidant drinks as long as they're made fresh. If white teeth are important to you, skip the black tea and drink a different color. We recommend a recipe we call *Tapple*, which is made with bioavailable, fresh, preferably organically-grown tea leaves that have been steeped for about four minutes, poured over ice and sweetened to taste with a splash of 100 percent organic apple juice (an antioxidant and slowly-absorbed glucose source). Other *BrightFoods* tea recipes can be found in Chapter Nine.

Given the blueberry, spinach, wheat, and tea examples, it's tempting to believe that heat or processing always reduces antioxidant bioavailability. Although this is a good general rule, there are some exceptions.

Lycopene Loves Processing

Tomatoes contain the antioxidant lycopene, which comes under the general heading "carotenoid." It gives them their color, and also makes watermelons and pink grapefruits red. A fresh one-ounce tomato contains less than one mg of lycopene, while an organically-grown tomato contains more. Surprisingly, when we process it up a notch, the numbers actually get better. An equivalent amount of tomato juice or soup contains three mg of lycopene. And when we kick it up further, we find that sauce or ketchup contains five mg and that tomato paste, the most processed of all, holds a whopping 16 mg of lycopene per ounce.

What about super-processed supplements? Studies have found that tomato juice and lycopene supplements work as antioxidants inside the body. When researchers looked at the concentration of pesticide residue on conventional tomatoes, they found that tomato puree has no more pesticide residue than a single unblanched and unprocessed tomato. But because organic tomato purees are also believed to be higher in other antioxidants, vitamin C, and polyphenols, and potentially lower in free radical-forming pesticide residue, purees made from organic tomatoes offer the most antioxidants.

So as you can see, "eating healthy" is a lot more complicated than experts would have us believe. When you get to Chapter Nine, note the recipes flagged with an A to see how the five *BrightFoods* mentioned above, along with the ones listed in Table 1, can be incorporated into easy-to-make recipes rich in antioxidants.

TABLE 1 – Other Foods Containing Antioxidants

Almond	Cinnamon	Peach
Apricot	Corn	Peanut Butter
Apple	Cucumber	Pear
Artichoke	Eggplant	Pea
Avocado	Garlic	Pepper
Banana	Grape	Plum
Beans	Kale	Potato
Beet	Kiwifruit	Raspberry
Black Pepper	Lettuce	Real Maple Syrup, Organic
Broccoli Floret	Melon	Scallion
Cabbage	Mustard	Strawberry, Organic
Cantaloupe	Nutmeg	Sunflower Seed
Carrot	Old Fashioned Oats	Turmeric
Cauliflower	Olive Oil	Walnut
Celery	Onion	Stone Ground Wheat Pasta
Cherry	Orange	Stone Ground Wheat Bread
Chocolate, Dark	Oregano	Zucchini

It can be complicated choosing the right foods, but with *BrightFoods*, you don't have to become a medical nutritionist or nutritional neuropsychiatrist. Just leave the shopping and cooking to us.

Chapter Summary

- Excited oxygen molecules called "free radicals" cause oxidative stress, which can corrode or rust brain hardware and software. Oxidative stress also plays a role in a variety of medical illnesses outside the brain, including cancer.
- Brain rust is associated with poor thinking, inattentiveness, slowed learning, mind-fog, memory loss, and decreased performance.
- Antioxidants in whole foods can behave differently than their processed or supplement forms.
- Just because an antioxidant displays free radical-zapping muscle outside the body doesn't necessarily mean that it will work as expected inside the body.
- Bioavailable antioxidants are free radical terminators that reduce oxidative stress and brain cell-rusting, and improve cell-networking and growth, focus, learning, memory, higher-order mental abilities, and performance.
- If you have to eat addictive meals with large amounts of protein, saturated fat and cheese, and therefore a big dose of free radicals, you can make the meal more medicinal by adding bioavailable antioxidant side dishes and a vitamin C supplement.

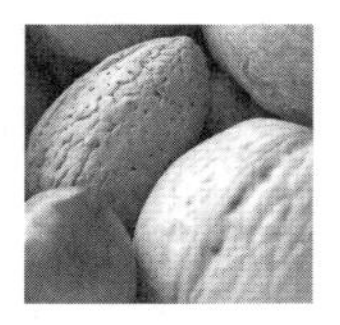

CHAPTER FOUR
Vital Oils Expand Brain Networking and Memory

Malnutrition n. A condition that comes from high-fat, low-fat, and wrong-fat diets
Obesity n. See "malnutrition"

The average American thinks fat is wicked because its high caloric content has been linked to overweight and obesity. By the end of this chapter you'll see a clear distinction between "bad fats," or those contributing to poor thinking, disease, and obesity, and "good fats" or "vital oils," which are essential to optimal learning, memory, mood, and performance.

The more you deprive yourself of vital oils, follow high-fat or low-fat diets, or rely on vital oils that aren't adequately absorbed or assimilated into your body, the dimmer you become. You also bulge and age more, and perpetuate an ongoing "vital oil deficiency" within brain cells and the body in general. Perhaps your cravings for fat-laden addictive foods like bacon, cheese, and ice cream emerge from your faltering brain crying for help due to its vital oil deficiency. But before you absorb a better understanding of vital oils, let's go back in the nutrition time-machine and see where our perception of "fats" went wrong.

In 1927, scientists first noticed that a deficiency in fat affects both growth and reproduction. This observation began a hunt for what they called "vitamin F." Researchers eventually found two: linoleic and linolenic acids. They referred to these as "essential fatty acids," since it was believed that the body needed to get them from foods in order to manufacture other key functional and energy-providing oils.

By the late 1970s, it was apparent that children who are deficient in linoleic acid develop severe skin problems, while those deficient in linolenic acid develop nervous problems. The discovery of linoleic and linolenic acids, along with their vital roles in health maintenance, showed for the first time that fat isn't just something to avoid, and that there's a "good" as well as a "bad" type of fat. This was big news, but the American public didn't really latch on to it.

Today there is a wealth of new research and information about how vital oils affect the brain and help us live brighter, longer, and happier lives, while bad fats are not only detrimental to the heart, but also to the brain. Let's take an aerial view of all fats.

The Ugly, the Bad, and the Good

When it comes to thinking well, there are three basic types of fats: ugly, bad, and good.

The ***ugly*** ones are "trans fatty acids," because they transform semi-wholesome oils into ones that are unhealthy. They're unnatural, and they cause disease. Trans fats are formed when manufacturers heavily process oils by adding hydrogen atoms at high pressures and temperatures, giving us that smooth creamy texture we love in margarine and other processed foods. This process is called "hydrogenation." Without hydrogenation, most vegetable oils wouldn't be creamy, and would oxidize or turn rancid. When consumed over time, hydrogenated oils impair brain cell networking, learning, memory, mood, and performance.

Some vegetable oils, like flaxseed, are especially subject to oxidation, and can turn unhealthy shortly after being pressed without any additional processing. Others, such as olive oil, are resistant to oxidation, and don't require hydrogenation to stay fresh and tasty, because they contain antioxidants.

Because trans fats have no nutritional value and can impair thinking, they aren't found in *BrightFoods* recipes.

The ***bad*** fats are the "saturated fats" found in meat, whole milk, butter, and cheese, and the "partially hydrogenated vegetable oils" found in margarine, mayonnaise, and oils such as canola, corn, and soybean. Relatively small quantities of saturated fat are found in lean meats, low fat milk, yogurt, and cheese.

Processed lower calorie vegetable oils, especially when used in deep frying, contribute to saturated fat deposits in the brain, and interfere with normal brain cell functioning. When bad fats dominate our diet over time, they contribute to impaired learning, memory, mood, and performance, and to obesity, disease, and aging. For this reason, when we see that the foods on our plates contain moderate to large amounts of bad fat, *BrightFoods* recommends off-setting the potential barrage of free radical formation and absence of antioxidant fire-power with healthier items. We can add a little vital oil to one of the side dishes, drip some on unburnt toast, or add some bioavailable antioxidant foods (see the chart from the last chapter) so we remain ahead in the war on free radicals.

The ***good*** fats are collectively called "vital oils." Seven sovereign oils more or less make up this constellation. They are the following acids:

- Linoleic, which turns into vital oil #2 (gamma linolenic), which turns into vital oil #3 (Arachidonic)
- Linolenic, which turns into EPA (eicosapentaenoic), which turns into DHA (docosahexaenoic)
- Oleic

Linoleic, linolenic, and oleic acids in their non-hydrogenated forms are all found in olive oil.

Now that we have introduced you to the Sovereign Seven, let's look at some ways the body benefits from vital oils.

What Good Are Vital Oils?

- They add flavor to food, reducing the need for salt.
- They help us absorb vitamins A, D, E, and K, making them bioavailable.
- They make up cell membrane structure, and are necessary for nutrients to move into and within cells (we call this ability "fluidity").
- They make substances that help fight impaired thinking, arthritis, blood clotting, inflammation and lupus, and prevent heart attacks and autoimmune diseases, as well as help stabilize the immune system.
- They're necessary for healthy hair and skin; if you're dependent on skin lotion, you're likely to be deficient in them.

- They aid sexual function.
- They monitor cholesterol metabolism.
- They help deter seizures.
- Shortages of them are sometimes associated with obesity, premature aging, and death.
- They make all living cells, especially brain cells, function and work with heightened efficiency.
- They may help reduce our appetite for bad fats, while at the same time improving learning, memory, mood, and performance.

These are most of the ways vital oils provide wellness from head to toe. Let's take a closer look at the role of vital oils in brain cells and the mind.

Vital Oils, Brain Cells, and the Mind

Before the turn of the twenty-first century, the link between vital oils and the mind was relatively controversial. Some scientists believed there was a link, while others thought it might be possible, and still others saw no connection. Most agreed that vital oils were not harmful when adults kept their consumption limited to around 15 to 20 percent of their total daily caloric intake. This safety statement applied strictly to vital oils, as opposed to ugly and bad fats, of course.

Still, while some clinical researchers had long been reporting anecdotal evidence of a link between vital oils and enhanced performance, the happy connection didn't get a lot of attention in the scientific community until recently. (On a personal note, I ate mashed potatoes using olive oil as gravy as far back as 1975, so I could focus better and have more energy while cramming for exams at Rutgers University.)

By the turn of this century, academic researchers were turning up more evidence of the association between vital oils and clear thinking, though there was still some controversy about it. Maybe some of these researchers hadn't yet taken the oils' bioavailability into consideration, or they may have used processed oils or an isolated vital oil in the absence of other food groups in their studies. And not one study looked at the association between thinking and the combination of bioavailable antioxidants, vital oils, smart proteins, and slowly-absorbed glucose that enhance it.

Nonetheless, a substantial amount of research is beginning to emerge showing the impact vital oils have on brain cell plasticity and thinking ability. Let's look at how each affects the mind, one player at a time.

Linoleic acid – Dietary linoleic directly influences brain cell structure. Numerous studies have linked linoleic to improved thinking in general, and learning and memory in particular. In addition, linoleic may be useful in treating depression and attention deficit hyperactivity disorder. Linoleic is chemically converted into gamma linolenic.

Gamma linolenic acid – A deficiency of this vital oil has been linked to attention deficit hyperactivity disorder, and it may improve learning and memory when present in adequate quantities. The molecular structure of gamma linolenic can be metabolically changed slightly, turning it into arachidonic acid.

Arachidonic acid – A deficiency of this vital oil has been linked to aging and attention deficit hyperactivity disorder. Some believe that arachidonic improves brain cell development, learning, and memory.

Linolenic acid – This vital oil directly influences the structure and function of different parts of the brain cell. Linolenic has been associated with decreased hyperactivity and improved behavior, including the ability to adapt to new situations. In addition, linolenic is known to improve thinking in general and attention, learning, memory, and pleasure perception in particular. Because animal sources of linolenic also seem to be medicinal, it might be useful for more vendors to enrich egg yolk with linolenic. Linolenic can chemically convert into EPA.

EPA – Eicosapentaenoic acid affects brain cell membranes and function. It's associated with improved brain cell development, attention, intelligence, learning, memory, and mood, and thinking in general. It may also improve behavior. EPA can chemically change into DHA; both are found in fish oil.

DHA – Docosahexaenoic, also known as "cervonic acid," influences brain structure and function, and has been associated with improved brain cell development, intellectual functioning, learning, memory, mood, and temperament in particular, and thinking in general. DHA may reduce defiant and hyperactive behavior. More evidence links DHA to improved thinking and behavior than to any other vital oil. Dietary DHA works best in the presence of adequate amounts of linoleic, gamma linolenic, arachidonic, linolenic, EPA, and oleic.

Oleic acid – Although it is made inside our brain, dietary sources of oleic are important, since oleic increases the ability of nutrients to move into, within and out of brain cells. It doesn't compete with the assimilation of linoleic and linolenic, and it's an antioxidant that helps keep linoleic and linolenic from spoiling or turning rancid. A few studies have reported a link between oleic and improved thinking.

The different fatty acids play different roles within our bodies to keep us healthy. This is how it works: Because they're so important to us, linoleic and linolenic become like the CEO and CFO of a Fortune 500 company, with unprocessed oleic functioning as their administrative assistant. So how does oleic acid make things happen for linoleic and linolenic? Oleic acid becomes concierge par excellence once it gets off the protein or carbohydrate shuttle by acting as a door-keeper and helping the bosses—linoleic and linolenic—get into brain cells. Without standing in their way or competing with them for entrances, it opens doors for them—that is, it increases their ability to permeate cells. Increased brain cell fluidity makes it easier for the linoleic and linolenic to get in and get to work. Researchers in the past may have overlooked this concierge connection, skewing test results that used linoleic or linolenic alone without their natural partner, oleic.

Oleic also maintains its antioxidant strength inside the brain to a large extent, and along with the other antioxidants in olive oil, stands bodyguard to both linoleic and linolenic, protecting them from oxidation or turning rancid. With these antioxidant preservatives, olive oil helps keep linoleic and linolenic from getting "fired" by the oxidation process.

Also, oleic is thought to replace harmful saturated fats in brain cells, and cells throughout the body. This is why olive oil, with the highest un-hydrogenated oleic to saturated fat ratio in Table 2, can help lower the overall saturated fat impact of a meal or snack. Beyond that, oleic packs an electron laser, and whacks free radicals as they drive by. For these and other reasons, oleic is more important to our diets than we previously thought.

So, all we have to do is ingest plenty of foods containing linoleic and linolenic acids, and we'll live smarter, happier and longer, right? As we explained in the section about antioxidants and their varying bioavailability, the answer isn't as simple as just taking in more vital oils. Living smarter, happier, and longer requires absorbing the Sovereign Seven and assimilating them in the right proportions, so they're bioavailable to our brain cells.

In other words, if we want to improve our thinking abilities, we need to consume bioavailable sources of vital oils. Just because a food or supplement contains "linolenic" or "fish oil" doesn't mean we are reaping its benefits. The secret to optimal bioavailability and clear thinking is consuming foods containing a certain ratio of vital oils.

The Right Ratio Yields the Right Results

Taking in large amounts of vital oils in foods and/or supplements doesn't necessarily mean that your brain cells can make good use of them. Linoleic and linolenic need to be ingested in a certain ratio to each other, or the two fatty acids compete with one another, and only one gets inside. This presents a challenge. Ingest too much linoleic oil, which half the vegetable oils in Table 2 contain, and a linolenic deficiency can result, increasing the likelihood of inflammation and blood clotting, and decreasing immune response.

On the other hand, take too much linolenic, which could happen if you had too much fish oil or fresh pressed flaxseed oil, and you'll reduce the absorption of linoleic, which can hurt the way brain cell membranes function and cancel any extra brightness you thought you were getting from your linolenic infusion.

When it comes to ideal absorption and bioavailability of vital oils and the way they're best distributed in the body, the correct ratio of linoleic to linolenic in the presence of unprocessed oleic seems to be what makes these two major players work optimally for brain cell energy and structure, and enhanced learning and memory.

TABLE 2 – Ratios of Linoleic to Linolenic and Ratios of Oleic to Saturated Fats in Common Oils

	Linoleic:Linolenic Ratio	Oleic:Saturated Fat Ratio
Butter Fat	1:1	1:2
Canola (Rapeseed) Oil	2:1	10:1
Beef Fat	2:1	1:1
Olive Oil	5:1	6:1
Lard Fat	6:1	1:1
Soy Oil	8:1	2:1
Chicken Fat	10:1	2:1
Flaxseed Oil	1:3	3:1
Corn Oil	30:1	2:1
Safflower Oil	76:1	1:1
Coconut Oil	4:0	1:11
Palm Oil	5:0	1:7
Peanut Oil	34:0	3:1
Sunflower Oil	68:0	2:1

When you read the chart, look for ratios of linoleic to linolenic in the 2:1 to 10:1 range. Nearly half of the oils in Table 2 fall there: They're canola oil, beef fat, olive oil, lard fat, soy oil, and chicken fat. Of these six, beef, lard, and chicken fat have little linoleic and linolenic value due to the unhealthy ratio of oleic to saturated fat. That leaves canola, soybean, and olive oil as possible contenders for the ideal bioavailability award. And canola and soybean oils are processed using hydrogen gas, high pressure, and high temperatures to keep them from spoiling; this partial hydrogenation may disturb the chemical structure and influence the bioavailability of both linoleic and linolenic in these oils.

What's left? Olive oil, with a linoleic to linolenic ratio of 5:1, in the middle of the range. In addition, olive oil is not partially-hydrogenated, because it contains natural antioxidant preservatives that keep the vital oils fresh and bioavailable, both outside and inside the body. For these reasons, the *BrightFoods*

"Bioavailable Vital Oils Award" goes to olive oil. And filtered olive oil is safe for cooking and baking, because it can be heated to 400 degrees F.

There are other unprocessed sources of vital oils, such as avocados and walnuts, but more are needed. *BrightFoods* is developing a 5:1 ratio of linoleic to linolenic-fortified peanut butter, similar to the efforts on behalf of infant formulas and eggs, and supplements. *BrightFoods* brings vital oils into school and work cafeterias, healthcare facilities and your home with 5:1 fortified meals and snacks in the sample menus and recipes (see Chapter Nine).

Vital oils and other medicinal foods—bioavailable antioxidants, smart proteins, and slowly-absorbed glucose—are like medicines. That is to say: too little is ineffective, and too much can be harmful.

Where Do They Go Once Inside?

As we mentioned, vital oils catch a ride on a protein or carbohydrate shuttle to get to where they are going. For this reason, eating olive oil with some smart protein such as free range chicken or slowly-absorbed glucose such as cucumber makes it more bioavailable than if olive oil or one of its components is taken alone. Also, the benefits of olive oil are reduced when taken with processed proteins such as delicatessen meats or soy, or with rapidly-absorbed glucose from fries. This could explain why a few studies looking at the connection between vital oils and smarts came up empty-handed.

Once inside the brain, some of the linoleic and linolenic acids from foods provide sustained energy, and do it better than saturated fats. Maybe that's why diets containing 15 to 20 percent vital oils provide added endurance, while diets rich in saturated fat provide added cushioning. While some of the linoleic and linolenic provides energy, another part serves as brick, mortar, and electrical wiring, and becomes part of the brain cell structure. As for gamma linolenic, arachidonic, EPA, and DHA coming from food sources, they're sucked up faster than the same substances when they're manufactured inside our bodies. Because vital oils give us enduring energy and become part of our brain hardware and all the other body cells, we probably get more fat that ends up as padding from a few fat-free rice cakes (because rapidly-absorbed glucose is stored as fat) than from a tablespoon of olive oil.

While we're still focused inside the body, let's look at why we don't really need to eat fish or take fish oil to get smarter.

We're All Pisces in One Way

Scientists used to believe that our bodies were incapable of making linoleic or linolenic, but it turns out that they can lengthen the shorter fatty acids found in green leafy vegetables into linoleic and linolenic. Researchers confirmed this when they found larger amounts of linoleic and linolenic present inside the body than they'd originally measured in the food before it was eaten. From this, they figured out that our bodies manufacture "home-made" linoleic, linolenic, and all their derivatives—EPA and DHA, or "fish oil," the same compound that's found in actual fish.

Although *BrightFoods* has no problem with children and adults having the occasional fish dish (more about fish in the next chapter), fish-eaters are not necessarily getting more brain food. They're also not necessarily smarter than those of us who make home-grown "fish oil" from avocado, greens, olive oil or walnuts.

We have learned enough to get to another fascinating part of nutritional neuropsychiatry: how brain cells "learn."

Brain Plasticity, Memory, and Learning

Did you ever wonder how information is stored in memory cells? Now that we have seen how vital oils become part of a brain cell's hardware, it's easier to imagine how learning, memory, and performance emerge from brain cells.

There is much evidence to suggest that "files" of information are stored inside brain cell circuits. To understand this, imagine that Oprah's about to conduct an interview on television, and the different lines of conversation she might take are the "files" stored in her head. It's easier to retrieve information from stored files and create files containing new information when brain cell membranes are made pliable by vital oils. When vital oils are abundant in brain cells, they're said to be "plastic," enabling new information files to be formed, stored, and retrieved. The place where information related to learning and memory is stored is likely to be the space between brain cell connections called synapses. When we regularly eat small amounts of bioavailable vital oils in combination with other foods, we keep our brains and synapses pliable and plastic, making it easier for us to learn and remember.

Vital oils are so important to great thinking ability that you'd almost expect a warning light on our bodies to go on whenever one of the Sovereign Seven reaches a dangerously low level.

The "Fat Addiction" Theory

We know that prescription medicines are either curative or habit-forming. Xanax, for example, can quiet the emotional discomfort of anxiety and worry for about four hours, and then promptly refunds one's misery, with interest. In contrast, we don't experience uncomfortable withdrawal symptoms when an antibiotic or some other curative medicine wears off. In addition, we desire more and more of an addictive medicine, while curative medicines don't trigger such a progression.

Earlier on, we described how addictive foods such as fries, burgers, chips, ice cream, and cookies rapidly go down our throats, and how we can find ourselves hunting for more after a short period of time. We're more likely to eat medicinal foods in moderation, however, and they help us maintain focus and enjoy sustained energy. Eating medicinal foods also permits us to move on to the next non-eating activity, and keep hunger away for hours. We clearly tend to crave and eat larger portions of some foods, such as saturated fat-containing cheese, while we don't crave or eat large portions of foods containing olive oil. No one knows why.

The "Fat Addiction" Theory holds that a chronic deficiency in vital oils alters our thoughts to such an extent that an alarm sounds in our mind, which we "hear" in the form of an urge or craving for fatty food. This fat-craving alarm distracts us from whatever we're doing in an instinctive attempt to correct the underlying vital oils deficiency. Hence, we venture out in pajamas late at night for a bacon double cheeseburger, chips, fries, microwavable macaroni and cheese, or a pint of ice cream. But because these bad fats do not correct the vital oil deficiency, our craving for fatty foods continues.

When we correct the vital oil deficiency, we help reduce our cravings for fatty foods. Thousands of people in my clinical practice have dimmed down their fat craving switch by gradually increasing olive oil consumption along with the other three *BrightFoods* medicinal food groups. But there can be more to a food's "addictive" properties than its fat content.

Many of us find ourselves eating cheese like we've been denying ourselves the pleasure for months, and we keep eating it even after we feel like a walking dairy case. The reason could go beyond a possible instinctive attempt to correct an underlying vital oils deficiency. Brace yourself, because those curds really do act like a drug.

Yes, opiate-like substances in milk can become concentrated in cheese. These calming chemicals, called casomorphins, are known to have a drug-like effect on the brain, and to be partly responsible for our inability to eat just a little cheese. Casomorphins have even been studied in relation to sudden infant death syndrome (SIDS).

Could there be more to "cheese addiction" than the urge to eat fat and opiates? You bet. Cheese contains an amphetamine-like protein called phenylethylamine, and a second stimulant by the name of glutamate. The combined effect of the fat, opiate, and stimulants may create the perfect chemistry for a love affair with cheese. Most people, addicted or not, want their minds to be sharp and calm. This is why heroin addicts "speedball," or mix heroin with cocaine to get a soothing and more focused effect, while cocaine addicts in withdrawal often drink beer to strike a better emotional balance.

Whether we have a problem with cheese or are in denial, *BrightFoods* has found a way to help us eat cheese "socially," and not to excess. We serve it up in got-to-have meals like pizza and macaroni and cheese with extra antioxidant, smart protein, slowly-absorbed glucose and of course, bioavailable vital oils.

Chapter Summary

- Not all fats make us overweight or compromise health and longevity.
- Vital oils are essential to normal body functions, especially in the brain.
- Vital oils assimilate into the body better under certain conditions, and in specified ratios. More of one is not better.
- Low-fat, low-calorie, and high-fat diets can contribute to vital oil deficiency, mind dysfunction, disease, premature aging, and being overweight.

- Olive oil and greens can each turn into "fresh, home-made fish oil" inside our bodies.
- Brain plasticity is maintained by vital oils, and helps form memory files responsible for learning.
- There may be an explanation as to why we are addicted to certain foods containing trans or bad fats, while no one to our knowledge habitually consumes copious amounts of medicinal foods such as olive oil.
- There is considerable evidence to suggest that vital oils improve learning, memory, mood, and performance without making us overweight.

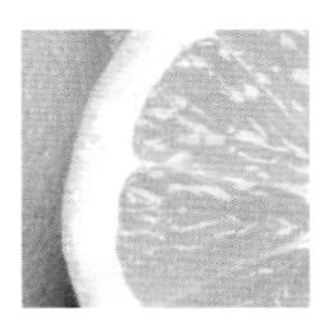

CHAPTER FIVE

Smart Proteins: Instant Messengers on the Brain-Wide Web

Though cheese, meat, eggs, and dairy are the most popular protein sources, they're not essential for great health. Vegans, as well as millions of Hindus and Buddhist and Orthodox Christian monks are living proof that minimally-processed grains, legumes, nuts, vegetables, and fruit provide enough protein to sustain productive lives. The recipes, medicinal ingredients and cooking methods mentioned in this book and the soon to be released *BrightFoods Cookbook* are designed to please not only them, but also people who have other preferences for how their protein is served up.

That's because protein is critical to health maintenance. When we burn protein from food to produce energy, we're left with exhaust composed of carbon dioxide, water, nitrogen, and free radicals. Some of the nitrogen waste is recycled much like blocks that snap into place to make brand new amino acids, while another portion becomes DNA, the blueprints of the body's master plan, and is stored inside each brain cell's nucleus. We also need the right amount of protein to have strong bones and immune systems; eating too little or too much can hinder the body's ability to defend itself against disease, and has been linked to osteoporosis.

How does it work? Protein chains are made up of nitrogen-containing links called "amino acids," and they come in two varieties. One type of amino acid link has branches in its structures that form a "y," which helps them more or less hook together to develop into muscle. Muscle is the second-largest energy storage site in the body, after adipose tissue, the fat that nestles in our midsection, though the energy stored in this form of muscle protein is rarely used by the body as fuel, unless it's starving. The other kind of amino acid link is shaped in a straight line to produce energy that's used by the brain (which also uses vital oils and slowly-absorbed glucose; we'll learn about this type in the next chapter).

When we consume foods containing protein, our bodies disassemble the protein chains into their many different amino acid link components. Many of the straight-shaped amino acid links, such as tryptophan, convert into neurotransmitters and serve as instant messengers on the brain-wide web. For example, tryptophan converts into serotonin. Each brain cell sends out an array of instant messengers, each type carrying and delivering a particular piece of information to other brain cells; in this case, serotonin tells brain cells not to worry and to be happy. In this way, brain cells chat with each other, and either convince the next brain cell to send the text message on to friends, or to stop sending that particular message.

There are countless brain cell-to-brain cell instant messages coming and going at any time, so that each brain cell listens to the equivalent of a few hundred phone conversations, while talking to a few hundred different people, all at the same time. What do the instant messages sound like? Something like "watch out!", "be afraid," "worry," "listen to that," "smile," "pay attention," "go to sleep," "wake up," "get a breakfast sandwich," "eat," "stop eating" or "relax." These neurotransmitters show how biology affects psychology and psychology affects biology, making brain biology and psychology one and the same. They're also the reason why some proteins are smart, because they can affect happiness, learning, memory, and performance. Let's look at some of the major neurotransmitters and "listen" to some of their messages.

Instant Messengers

Although we use protein to give us energy, form muscle, and make new amino acids and genetic material such as DNA, we'll focus here on how certain straight-shaped amino acids chemically convert into some of the main instant messengers in our brains. Probably the most well-known messengers are dopamine, norepinephrine, and serotonin (the one that prompts carefree feelings).

Tyrosine is an amino acid found in essentially all foods containing protein. Tyrosine turns into the instant messenger norepinephrine, which is important in controlling wakefulness, alertness, and learning. Norepinephrine can then chemically convert into dopamine, which is responsible for our emotional stability and the ability to pay attention and learn. Both norepinephrine and dopamine send instant messages onto other brain cells, promoting feelings of ambitiousness, attentiveness, drive, energy, and happiness. Dopamine is more responsible for sensations of ecstasy and bliss than norepinephrine.

Tryptophan is an amino acid that's found in essentially all protein-containing foods. There are higher concentrations of it in warm milk, though eggs and beans also contain tryptophan. As we mentioned, the body converts tryptophan into the instant messenger serotonin, which sends instant messages to other brain cells that make us feel soothed, patient, and serene. This is why consuming a large amount of turkey and other foods rich in tryptophan reduces anxiety and induces sleep. Besides regulating mood, serotonin is also important for optimal learning and memory.

Table 3 summarizes how instant messaging changes when alcohol and cocaine are being abused, or when someone is obese and abusing food, and tryptophan levels get too low. This is an association that I studied with my research colleagues, Dr. Mark S. Gold and Dr. Jeffrey Jonas, in 1986. All three "addictions" deplete dopamine and norepinephrine formed from tyrosine, making a person feel lazy, tired, bored, confused, and forgetful. In the same way, these three addictions are associated with serotonin depletion, which can make an individual irritable, worried, anxious, intolerant, overwhelmed, and unable to sleep. In short, protein and the instant messengers into which it transforms directly affect the way we feel, behave, and learn.

TABLE 3 – Neurotransmitters and Nutrition

Instant Messenger	Depleted in Alcohol & Cocaine Abuse	Depleted in Obesity	Effect of Depletion on Mood	Amino-Acid Building Block	Occurs Naturally In
Dopamine, Norepin-ephrine	YES	YES	No energy or drive; poor focus; depression	Tyrosine	Poultry, lean meat, eggs, peas, green beans, wheat, oats, yogurt, milk
Serotonin	YES	YES	Agitation, impatience, insomnia	Tryptophan	Turkey, meat, eggs, beans, nuts, seeds, yogurt, milk

Adapted from *THE 800-COCAINE Book of Drug and Alcohol Recovery*, 1990

Now that we have a basic understanding of instant messaging, let's take it to the next level to appreciate how rocket science pales compared to brain science. But don't worry—we'll just be examining a few other important instant messengers.

More Amino Acids and Their Messages

There are 20 different amino acids in the body, but only some become instant messengers.

Glutamic acid, or glutamate, sends some of the most "exciting" messages a brain cell can receive. You may recognize "glutamate" from monosodium glutamate, or MSG, a flavor enhancer often added to some restaurant and processed foods. I can just hear the heavily-processed, bagged, boxed, canned-food lovers say "See, MSG is natural, so it's got to be good for you." I respond to that by pointing out how arsenic is also a natural and curative medicine when it's taken in physician-prescribed tiny amounts.

As we'll discuss in the chapter on additives and toxins, it's believed that a mild to moderate amount of glutamate makes the amino acid a useful stimulating messenger to learning and memory. Take too much, though—and glutamate naturally occurs in excess in processed soy, whey, and cheese—

and glutamic acid, along with its by-product, glutamine, can turn into a brain cell toxin. That means that ingesting too much glutamate feels great for a short while, but then brain cells can become excited to the point of brown-out and even death, as they're gunned down with the same mercilessness with which free radicals pummel cells.

Glycine is an essential amino acid like glutamate that also has a stimulating effect, but of a different variety. Glycine may play a role in modulating our motivation and recall. However, it does not seem to be a major player in mood regulation, memory that's used for problem solving, or attentiveness.

Gamma aminobutyric acid, or GABA, is the main fast-acting sedative in the brain. It is chemically derived from glutamate. Medicines that increase GABA's action include antiepileptics, sedatives, and anti-anxiety agents; alcohol has the same effect. A disrupted GABA system causes emotional sensitivity, poor impulse control, impaired concentration, stress, depression, irritability, and anxiety. GABA is related to memory, mood, thought, and spatial learning—that is, the ability to understand how objects occupy space (for example, realizing that a six-foot couch will not fit along a four-foot wall).

Acetylcholine is made from choline, which is present in large amounts in egg yolks, legumes, and grains. There is strong evidence linking acetylcholine to attention, learning, memory, thinking, and behavior-related messages. Together, dopamine and a particular type of acetylcholine are crucial to heightening attentiveness.

Adenosine is a precursor to DNA, but it is also an instant messenger. Adenosine plays a big role in the psychological affects of caffeine, and is also thought to affect sleep, awakening, learning, and memory.

Endorphins induce physical and emotional pain relief much like prescription pain pills do. These heroin-like messengers elevate mood and well-being, and make it easier to cope. They can also have amnesic and anxiety-reducing properties, and they enhance performance and appetite.

Cholecystokinin, or CCK, improves attention, learning, and memory. It communicates with the intestine on a daily basis, and inside the brain, CCK decreases appetite, anxiety, panic, and stress levels.

There are many other known instant messengers, some of them hormones, and it's suspected that many more are yet to be discovered. Our brain contains a virtual pharmacy of mind medicines which send information through the brain-wide web, ranging from mood elevators, anti-anxiety agents and pain-killers to attention, learning, memory, and performance accelerators. We need to replenish the ones that come from amino acids by eating smart proteins, so that about 20 to 30 percent of our daily intake of calories comes from them. If you're good in math and want to figure out your approximate *daily protein requirement*, multiply 0.7 gm of protein times half your body weight. For example, a 140-pound individual should eat about:

70 X 0.7 = 49 grams or 2 ounces of protein per day

Table 4 shows some foods that are great sources of smart protein when eaten with the right amount of bioavailable antioxidants, vital oils, and slowly-absorbed glucose.

TABLE 4 – Smart Protein Sources When Minimally Processed and, Ideally, Organic

Animal Sources	Plant Sources
Brighter Fish	Breads made of Stone Ground Whole Wheat
Chicken	Dried Peas
Eggs	Dried Beans
Game Meat	Grains in the SA List, Appendix III
Lean Cuts of Beef	Nuts, Unsalted
Lean Cuts of Lamb	Peanut Butter
Lean Cuts of Pork	Seeds
Lean Cuts of Veal	Vegetables
Low Fat Milk & Plain Yogurt	Wild Rice
Turkey	

In case you're wondering how vegans get their protein, here are some ways:

- Legumes, lentils, and slowly-absorbed rice
- Leafy vegetables, sesame seeds, and slowly-absorbed wheat and other whole grains
- Slowly-absorbed corn, peas, and other produce, and nuts

BrightFoods suggests limiting the amount of highly-processed proteins in your diet. Besides delicatessen and canned meats, there are basically three highly-processed protein sources: soy, whey, and cheese.

Soy protein comes in many forms, including soy bacon substitute, cheese, diet bars, hydrolyzed protein, ice cream, milk, protein isolate, salad dressings, sauce, tofu, and veggie burgers. You can also find it in many power bars, and health and fitness drinks and powders. Don't get me wrong; as the developer of a "zero cholesterol" cookbook in 1984 that used an abundance of processed soy products as ingredients, I loved the stuff. I was right up there with the soy-loving Californians, but hid the fact, being a Jersey boy.

It wasn't until 2001, when I began writing *The Mood Diet* (a book that elaborated on my 1985 "Sobriety Diet") that I changed my tune regarding soy. I knew soy products. Soy products were friends of mine. And processed soy is no medicinal food.

Soy beans are very high in protein. But the first step in processing them involves chemical treatment and heating, which breaks down protein and releases glutamate. The more soy is processed, the more glutamate is freed. Subsequently, a glutamate imbalance can occur in the brain when highly processed soy is used in excess. Over time, this causes brain cells to brown-out or be excited to death.

This interferes with optimal thinking abilities. In addition, soy infant formulas have been linked to aluminum brain cell toxicity (Fernandez-Lorenzo JR, et al; Greger JL, et al; Koo WW, et al; van der Voet GB, et al), and processed soy has been linked to attention deficit and behavioral problems in children, as well as learning disabilities, manganese toxicity (Cockell KA, et al; Collipp PJ, et al; Golub MS, et al) and memory impairment.

Outside the brain, processed soy has been associated with lessening the nutritional impact of foods, bone brittleness, coughing, fluoride poisoning, impaired digestion of nitrogen, kidney stone formation, stunted growth, thyroid tumors, and pancreatic cancer, which is on the rise in the US. Soy allergies are becoming more common. Signs and symptoms include diarrhea, facial swelling, fainting, hives, increased perspiration, shortness of breath, sneezing, and, rarely, anaphylaxis.

Soy often appears on ingredient labels as "hydrolyzed plant," "textured plant" or "vegetable protein." In any form, you don't need to be concerned about eating smaller amounts of soy, since it's found in a large variety of processed foods. But it can be risky business to take in too much processed soy daily in the form of "complete nutrition" drinks, which are often used in health care facilities by the debilitated and the mature. And it may be unnecessary to eat any, given the large variety of smarter protein sources available. For more information on medicinal drinks and foods for the debilitated, you'll be able to consult *BrightFoods for Cancer*, the next book in this series.

Also, because the regular use of soy has never been proven to be safe for all organ systems, and the few medicinal claims made for it remain unsubstantiated, many pediatricians advocate that soy infant formula be dispensed *by prescription only*. Perhaps "complete nutrition" formulas for adults should follow the same route.

Whey, the watery part of milk that separates from the curds, is favored among body builders who believe that it enhances muscle mass. But whey and other amino acid supplements haven't received the nod from scientists who've performed well-controlled studies on them. Whey's health benefits are also not well-established. The protein sources listed in Table 4 may do just as good a job as whey, if not better, in building body mass and general health. Another reason for avoiding excess dietary protein is that, if it's not used for energy, it's stored as fat instead of building muscle mass.

We should only consume recommended amounts of protein along with other medicinal foods. Balanced amounts of bioavailable antioxidants, vital oils, smart proteins, slowly-absorbed glucose, resistance training, and aerobic exercise will make us big without the help of whey, or branched-chain amino acid supplements.

There is also evidence to suggest that some damaging free glutamate, released during whey processing, rises to high levels in the brain after we drink excess amounts of whey-based body-building shakes. One study found no increase in the presence of glutamate in muscle, the liver, and the mucous found in the intestinal tract, but it didn't measure changes in free glutamate in relation to brain cell toxicity and thinking ability.

So how does glutamate form in whey? Enzymes are added to milk, and the mixture is heated in order to separate the curds and whey, and glutamate is formed during this process. After that, whey is further processed and dried, possibly generating even more glutamate. Finally, there's additional processing to make whey protein isolate, freeing still more.

Another reason why we don't count whey as a smart protein is because excess heating may alter many of the amino acids in it, rendering them more bio-*unavailable*. Lastly, studies suggest an association between whey protein and impaired regulation of the body's defenses or immune responses, changes in motivation and the ability to remember, as well as mineral toxicity and blood-thinning activity.

Cheese, preferably low fat and low sodium, should be reserved for major meals such as *BrightFoods* pizza, macaroni and cheese, or lasagna. There are many reasons to believe that it's unnecessary, unhealthy for the brain and body, and habit-forming to eat too much cheese. Take it from a recovering cheese addict: Cheese belongs at the top—that is, the smallest part—of the *BrightFoods* Pyramid (Appendix I), because the wonderful stuff contains way too much mind-fogging, disease-causing fat. Cheese is also short on smart protein, because it can also produce excess mind-disrupting glutamate. Its relatively high amounts of saturated fat and salt can tax the heart, as well. And under certain circumstances, its high salt content can even lead to stomach cancer.

We have looked at smart proteins and not-so-smart proteins. That leaves fish somewhere in the middle.

It's Smart Protein When You Know How to Fish

We question whether it's a good idea to follow the American Heart Association's recommendation of eating at least two servings per week of fish. Why? Because fish is a food that's easily contaminated with free radical-, brain rust-forming mercury, and disease-causing dioxins such as polychlorinated biphenyls (PCBs). These substances may be toxic to brain cells, and contraindicated in children and pregnant moms. Smart protein is readily available from many other foods, and "fish oil" can be made in our bodies from olive oil and certain vegetables.

Over the years, my clients have asked, "What fish can my children and I eat, and how often?" This is tough to answer, because as in most areas of health and nutrition, no one has taken an adequate consumer-friendly leadership role. Instead, all we have is a plethora of fad diet fairy tales. So *BrightFoods* has developed the first detailed guidelines to fish consumption. The guidelines are very conservative because, as we mentioned earlier with respect to the good monks and Hindus, fish consumption is not essential to life. Lean meats and other protein sources may carry a lower toxicity potential. This is especially painful to swallow for a person who still barbeques ten-minute-old tuna, Wahoo, or Mahi Mahi fillets medium-well by the waters between Palm Beach and the Bahamas.

The good and not-so-good news is summarized in Table 5. If you want a Ph.D. in ichthyology, start by going to "Fish School" in Appendix II.

TABLE 5 – Summary of BRIGHTER Fish

Species	For Adults	For Children and Pregnant Moms
Shrimp	No frequency limit	No frequency limit
Whiting	No frequency limit	No frequency limit
Flounder	Twice weekly	Once biweekly
Talapia	Twice weekly	Once biweekly
Whitefish	Once weekly	Once monthly
Lobster	Once weekly	Once monthly
Chilean Bass	Once biweekly	Not recommended
Halibut	Once biweekly	Not recommended
Swordfish	Once monthly	Not recommended

It's fine to break out the broiler, but pick your fish wisely, cook to perfection and be prepared to balance out the meal with antioxidants.

The "Protein Addiction" Theory

I once wondered, especially after one of my annual six-week vegan runs, why my car drove itself, as if by wizardry, to a place like Outback Steakhouse while I was in a carnivore-crazed and steak-infatuated trance. What's up with that?

There are many reasons why meat in general, and beef in particular, may be habit-forming. One is that protein may increase insulin in the body more than certain carbohydrates, and that cell sensitivity to glucose also increases. This means that when we eat protein, more of that good-feeling glucose juice gets inside our brain cells. Reason One for the "Protein Addiction" hypothesis, therefore, is the feeling of well-being that eating meat causes. Reason Two may be the high concentrations of saturated fat, which when burned, generate energy and endurance. The last factor possibly contributing to the addictive nature of meat involves its ability to release soothing opiates via insulin. Therefore meat can be addictive, because it contains the magical drug combination of two stimulants and an opiate, prompting a soothing but alert state of mind. Perhaps the scientists who have localized protein craving to at least one area of the brain would agree.

Let's look at the most addictive food of all. Drum-roll please: Enter chocolate. Most of you probably won't find it hard to believe that it's thought to possess the largest number of addictive food properties. Chocolate contains three stimulants: caffeine; theobromine (Theo is the Greek word for "God"), which produces a "godly" feeling in humans, but can cause disease in dogs; and the amphetamine-like phenylethylamine, from the amino acid link phenylalanine. Chocolate has a calming and sedating opiate effect, because the opiate blocker naloxone cuts chocolate cravings. Finally, a fifth substance increases the amount of anandamide, a relative of the active ingredient in marijuana, found in the brain. Holy mackerel! Three stimulants, a minimal opiate and pot-like effects. It's no wonder why we can't stay out of Godiva Chocolatier.

But have no fear. We can eat chocolate once we know the detoxification plan (no whining, please). The sixth addictive component, whole milk, is what makes milk chocolate way more addictive than dark chocolate, and that makes detoxification from milk chocolate a snap. While a fling with milk chocolate that's high in rapidly-absorbed glucose feels like it can go on forever, when we eat dark chocolate, we have what we want and then we're done. And dark chocolate is healthier, and contains useful antioxidants.

A Brighter Ride:

What did the dopamine say to the endorphin?
Answer: Snap out of it!

Chapter Summary

- Protein comes from food sources besides meat, eggs, and cheese.
- Protein turns into neurotransmitters that send messages 24/7 across the brain-wide web.
- It's fine to occasionally eat soy, whey, and cheese.
- When consumed frequently, meat, cheese, and milk chocolate can act in the brain like addictive drugs.
- Slowly-absorbed breads, cereals, grains, legumes, vegetables, seeds, nuts, and fruit provide protein for vegans, so they can replenish their instant messengers.
- Chicken, turkey, lean meats, eggs, low fat milk and plain yogurt, game meat, and certain fish provide smart protein which can improve attention, learning, memory, mood, and performance.

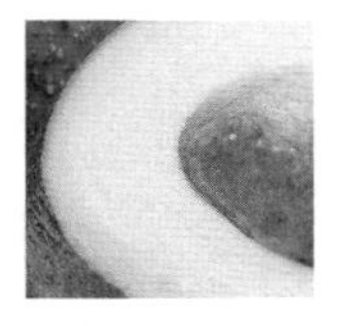

CHAPTER SIX
Slowly Absorbed Glucose: High-Speed Access to Well-Being

Synonyms for "low-carb:" tired, hungry, overweight

Brain cells need a steady and sustained flow of not only oxygen, but glucose, too. Take away either one, and it's not possible to learn, think, plan or solve problems. Though having too much oxygen or glucose can harm brain cells, having too little can be fatal. Unlike oxygen, however, blood glucose levels in the brain come directly from the food we eat, which we can monitor.

Glucose behaves like a medicinal food under certain dietary circumstances, and as an addictive food in others. Unfortunately, the popular classification of carbohydrates as either "simple" or "complex" hasn't helped us to understand which foods lead to obesity. By the end of this chapter, you should be better able to tell when glucose might act as a medicinal food and improve thinking, and when it might act as an addictive food, jamming up the ability to think, and leading to carb cravings later on. For our purposes, we're grouping glucose-containing foods into three descriptive categories:

- Slowly-absorbed, or SA glucose-carbohydrates that provide enduring energy and properties for maintaining ideal weight
- Moderately-absorbed, or MA glucose-carbs that contribute to fluctuations in energy, mood, and disease, and to being overweight
- Rapidly-absorbed, or RA glucose-carbs that provide short bursts of energy followed by fatigue, moodiness, carbohydrate-craving, and hunger, and lead to obesity, diabetes and other serious illnesses

We classify glucose in this way because research, as well as my own clinical experience, leads me to believe that it behaves as a medicinal food when it's absorbed slowly, and as an addictive food when it's absorbed at a moderate-to-rapid rate. Table 6 lists some examples of each, and Appendix III offers a more comprehensive view.

TABLE 6 – Comparison of Rapidly, Moderately, and Slowly-Absorbed Glucose Sources

Rapidly-Absorbed Glucose	Moderately-Absorbed	Slowly-Absorbed Glucose
Bagel (ef)	Angel Hair Pasta (ef)	Apple Juice, Unsweetened
Bran Flakes	Basmati Rice	Bagels (BF)
Cheerios	Bran Muffin (ef)	Bread (BF)
Corn Chips	Brown Rice	Chips (BF)
Corn Flakes	Coca Cola	Cookies (BF)
English Muffin (ef)	Cranberry Juice	English Muffins (BF)
Fruit Roll-Ups	Frosted Flakes	Kellogg's Complete
Gatorade	Granular or Table Sugar	Maple Syrup (fake or organic)
Pretzels (ef)	Hamburger Bun	Muffins (BF)
Raisin Bran	Life Cereal	Old Fashioned Oats
Rice Crispies	Linguini, Thin (ef)	Pizza Crust (BF)
Total Cereal	Rye Bread (ef)	Stone-Ground Wheat Flour
White or Enriched Flour	Special K	Whole Wheat Macaroni (ad)
Whole Wheat Bread (ef)	Whole Grain Bread (ef)	Zone Breakfast Cereal

ef – made with processed enriched flour and/or whole wheat flour

BF – *BrightFoods* recipes contain only SA glucose ingredients

ad – cooked al dente or medium

This table was extrapolated and adapted from Foster-Powell K, Holt SH, Brand-Miller JC, International table of glycemic index and glycemic load values. *Am J Clin Nutr.* Jul;76(1):5-56, 2002

There's been a lot of controversy over the past few decades about the effects of glucose on thought and behavior. Most of the studies done before the year 2000 concluded that high blood glucose levels had no significant impact on a child's thinking ability, behavior or performance. At the time, though, scientists weren't aware of the different absorption rates among various glucose-containing food sources, and most studies focused on the relationship between the foods and childhood hyperactivity.

Over the past few years, however, many scientists have come to the conclusion that glucose is indeed the food most often associated with changes in the ability to think. A theory that has gradually gained credence is that certain glucose-containing foods contribute to *sustained* glucose levels in the brain, which is believed to be beneficial to thinking, while others contribute to *fluctuations* in brain glucose levels, which likely hurts the ability to think.

Before we explore the rationale behind this further, let's look at why researchers think glucose-containing foods and drinks, such as soda, might be so popular.

Glucose Is a Star

No one knows exactly why we love glucose, or why we often behave like drug-abusers around foods high in rapidly-absorbed glucose, such as bread, cake, cookies, donuts, and fries. Researchers do say that glucose is the brain's main fuel source, guzzled up inside subcellular generators called mitochondria to provide feel-good energy we can draw on quickly. Without this constant flow of energy from glucose, our brain cells don't perform well, and it's more difficult to think. Brain cells rely on it to function, just like our computers require electricity. In the same way, our brain's hardware and software work best with a steady uninterrupted flow of glucose, even while we're sleeping.

Some research suggests that our brain cells and ability to think clearly don't function well when glucose levels are both too low and too high. Even people who boast that they "eat healthy" might be surprised after reviewing Appendix III, and seeing how the foods they eat don't insulate them from glucose lows and highs. Regardless, it's becoming clear that a relatively constant "110-glucose power source" may work best to help us keep our thinking light switches on and shining bright.

Perhaps glucose level dips and surges contaminated older research results that looked into the link between glucose, behavior and thinking. Studies completed over the past few years, however, show an emerging recognition of the association between glucose, better thinking and feeling well. It's now believed that glucose helps improve brain cell reorganization and networking. Moreover, these improvements in brain cell plasticity may link glucose to a host of benefits: better learning, memory storage and retrieval, conscious awareness, mood, calming in infants, and longer lives for brain cells.

Many of us love glucose because it's the perfect recipe for learning, remembering, and feeling well, and helps us stay calm and alert. But this is only true if it comes from the right food sources. The glucose found in old-fashioned oats, for example, behaves like a prescription antidepressant, while glucose from a candy bar gives its consumer ups and downs similar to those associated with cocaine.

Let's look at both extremes, beginning with how too much glucose, too fast, can affect our thinking.

Rapidly-Absorbed Glucose and Power Surges

Most studies examining how thought is affected by high blood glucose, or "hyperglycemia," have been either poorly-controlled or focused on untreated diabetic patients. Nevertheless, they can indicate how too much glucose in the blood affects brain cells and thinking ability. (Note: They may not parallel what happens when people without diabetes experience milder glucose power surges.)

Based on these studies, many researchers suggest a link between hyperglycemia and impaired thinking, dementia, Alzheimer's, and other neurodegenerative diseases, mood disturbances, coordination problems, and brain aging. Taken along with other findings, we may conclude that milder or "mini" surges in glucose levels also contribute to changes in learning, memory, mood, performance, and brain cell aging in otherwise healthy people of all ages.

In addition, mini glucose surges in adults may cause temporary energy boost and relaxed feelings, while in some children, as with stimulant and sedative medicines, mild hyperactivity may occur. I can attest from my experiences on a bus in 1965 to the unhealthy but common practice of pumped-up varsity wrestlers popping scores of "pep pills," or glucose tablets, on an absolutely empty stomach. A shared placebo effect can get only partial credit for these students consistently becoming hyperactive.

But that's all we have—anecdotal evidence. It's still possible, though, that mini glucose power surges in non-diabetic people hurt thinking and performance in a manner that's similar to the way diabetic patients suffer from these symptoms.

What we know for certain is that brain glucose surges of any magnitude are often followed by glucose crashes. This happens most often when eating foods that contain rapidly-absorbed glucose. Highly-processed foods, including many breakfast cereals and whole wheat bread that's not stone ground, turn into glucose straight away, and are rapidly absorbed into the blood, causing glucose surges, and probably some degree of short-lived well-being. We believe that this may be why some people love the Atkins plan—they initially feel better not because they're eating a diet heavy in proteins and fat, but because they're shunning the moderate and rapidly-absorbed glucose-containg carbs and the glucose crashes they create.

The belief is that once the 110-glucose surge protector has been tripped in the brain, a siren sounds that responds to the uneasy situation by releasing insulin. Insulin, the concierge that opens cell doors for glucose, helps glucose get inside brain cells, and stores excess glucose it can't process as fat. At times, however, insulin is over-enthusiastic, and instead of lowering the blood glucose level to normal, it may actually allow the blood glucose level to go down too far, and cause a mini dip in the brain cell glucose level. So there may be a clear cause and effect chain of events: We eat foods containing rapidly-absorbed glucose, we experience a power surge, the insulin we produce in reaction over-manages, and a mini dip results, slowing us down and making it harder to think clearly.

Ironically, the low fat foods craze plays a role in causing glucose swings, and contributes to the current overweight, obesity and diabetes epidemic. In the absence of fat or oil, glucose surges more rapidly in the blood, and excess glucose changes into fat. For example, plain rice cakes have relatively low calories, and most people would probably believe that several of them eaten together provide less glucose to be stored as fat than one that's been topped with peanut butter. But the reverse may actually be true. The one topped with peanut butter has far more calories than a bunch of plain rice cakes, but because the plain bunch of rice cakes provide glucose in the absence of vital oils, they could, in theory, provoke a rapid rise in glucose levels, causing more to be stored as fat. Thirty minutes later, the resulting power dip can trigger a desire to eat again.

In contrast, very little, if any, of the higher-calorie rice cake topped with peanut butter ends up as fat, because the oil in peanut butter converts the RA rice cake into an SA in the stomach. The combination provides sustained energy, and suppresses hunger for up to two hours. This is another example of how low fat and low calorie diets offer the illusion of healthy eating, but in reality lead to something like malnutrition.

Brown-Outs

Let's look at the other end of the spectrum: low glucose levels that lead to impaired thinking. Again, the worst case scenario would be when someone suffers from mismanaged diabetes, and has dangerously low levels of glucose, or "hypoglycemia." Investigators have found that hypoglycemia affects brain cells, and causes problems with brain cell networking. It also hinders attentiveness, processing information gained through hearing and the ability to complete complex tasks and thoughts. It can lead to depression and energy loss, poor memory and mood, and even make simple tasks difficult.

Some believe that in non-diabetics, an over-reaction to insulin may lead to a mini dip in glucose levels, making them feel as though they're hungry. Even our moms intuitively knew, as they shouted "Don't eat that or you'll spoil your dinner" in the late afternoon, that glucose consumption is the number one short-term appetite suppressant. We believe that hunger is the brain's alarm, and that it sounds when any one of the four medicinal food tanks—the ones for antioxidants, vital oils, smart proteins, and especially glucose—is running on empty.

Perhaps the loudest hunger alarm of all rings out after a glucose shortage induces a brain cell brown-out. These low levels of energy-producing glucose may be behind the hunger, carbohydrate cravings, and varying degrees of attention deficit, forgetfulness, uneasiness, and poor commission of tasks that follow. Our minds switch from focusing on the task before us to thinking about how happy we'll be once we have the next carbohydrate snack in hand. The next time you eat a bowl of rapidly-absorbed cereal with skim milk, see if you can go even 45 minutes before your alarm starts up. Or take a critical look at how well you can think after starting your morning off with coffee and Splenda and drinking diet cola all day, shopping for dinner and then waiting in the Express Check-Out line behind a guy with 25 big items. By then, a serious brown-out can cause so much hunger that you feel impatient, intolerant, and irritable.

Few studies have examined the addictive nature of foods containing rapidly-absorbed glucose. So what is it about bread, candy, cereal, chips, cookies, donuts, and fries that make us keep coming back for more, even though we know they're not "health foods"?

The "Rapidly and Moderately Absorbed Glucose Addiction" Theory

When we think of bananas, cucumbers, wild rice, sourdough bread, old-fashioned oatmeal, and other foods containing slowly-absorbed glucose, we recall that for the most part, none of them keep calling us back for more. Now, let's focus on cookies and chips, foods that contain rapidly-absorbed glucose. Consider how fast we eat them, and how we crave more shortly thereafter. And what about snack time? Do you leave a few jelly beans or some popcorn for later? What is it about an apple or a few olives that is more than enough for us, while an entire box of Wheat Thins is not? Could it be an addiction to rapidly-absorbed glucose?

Here is how we believe it works: Slowly-absorbed glucose is not habit-forming, because it provides sustained glucose to brain cells for a few hours without causing power surges or brown-outs. On the other hand, rapidly-absorbed glucose is highly addictive, and moderately-absorbed glucose is addictive for at least three reasons. First, RA and MA glucose immediately provide a quick energy fix for the uneasy feelings associated with brown-outs. Consuming either is a reliable way to take our mood and level of attentiveness from zero to 60 in a few seconds. Second, RA and MA glucose may be associated with power surges that are indirectly involved in the release of natural heroin-like drugs. These make adults feel a short-term calmness and serenity, though in some children, it has the opposite effect. The third reason may be because power surges have been associated with increased levels of serotonin, a natural antidepressant.

But that is not the end of the story, because "withdrawal" symptoms begin about 40 minutes after polishing off the RA and MA. These include fatigue, uneasiness, and lack of motivation, the products of brain cell brown-outs. Collectively, we call this feeling "hunger," and what comes next is often a craving for the next fix on the RA glucose rollercoaster.

Happily, we don't have to go to rehabilitation for RA glucose addiction. There are ways to take back control of our eating habits, and increase our thinking ability, performance, feelings of well-being, and longevity.

A Slowly-Absorbed Glucose Workshop

So how do we get the right amount of SA glucose flowing through our brains as constantly and evenly as oxygen, without getting power surges or brown-outs?

We believe that part of the permanent solution is to eat meals in which 60 percent of the calories provided come from slowly-absorbed glucose; people who are physically active should take in an even higher percentage. This should keep our brain cells and minds humming at top efficiency, while we achieve and maintain our ideal weights. We don't necessarily have to make major changes in the meals we prefer as much as we need to monitor the ingredients in them. *BrightFoods* has developed recipes for our favorite dishes and snacks that substitute medicinal carbohydrates for addictive ones. Let's look at a few examples.

Pizza – Most pizza crusts are made with white flour. But this strips them of antioxidants and fiber, and makes them a major source of rapidly-absorbed glucose, potentially leading to power surges and brown-outs that create cloudy thinking. This in turn may make it tough for us to limit ourselves to just one or two slices, as we struggle to raise our energy levels. Glucose from crust absorbs faster when it's in low fat pizza, too, so there's no benefit to scrimping on those calories.

Changing the main ingredient in the crusts to 100 percent stone ground whole wheat flour turns ordinary white pizza crust into a more complete and balanced food in itself. It contains slowly-absorbed glucose, antioxidants, smart proteins, natural fiber, and more naturally-occurring vitamins. This crust meets the call for more whole grains in our diet. And while some bakers add moderately-absorbed granular sugar to their crust, we add slowly-absorbed organic maple syrup to ours, plus a little olive oil. This combination of ingredients can generate energy and stifle hunger for hours.

If you're not eating our pizza or making your own, you can improvise. Before eating store-bought, thin crust pizza, eat a garden salad topped with olive oil and sliced hardboiled egg, bean salad or poultry mini-burgers (recipe in Chapter Nine), and 500 mg of vitamin C. Also try topping each slice with a teaspoon of olive oil, leaving the crust's edge for the birds. This combination of ingredients will slow down the rate at which you absorb the store-bought pizza, making it healthier. There may also be leftover pizza.

Bread is another carb favorite, consumed in the form of toast in the morning, sandwiches at lunch, and as a side-dish with dinner. As with pizza crust, most bread is made of white flour, or "whole wheat flour." "Whole wheat flour," surprisingly, remains a source of rapidly-absorbed glucose, because it is a blend of highly processed flour that has been bleached. Our bread ingredients are similar to those in our pizza crust, and that can make our bagels, bread, dinner rolls, English muffins, hamburger buns, hot dog rolls, sub rolls, and wraps more beneficial to clear thinking than most conventional bread recipes. We use similar basic ingredients to make our buns, cakes, cookies, muffins, and pretzels, converting what some consider "junk food" into food that helps you "eat right."

People who do not enjoy baking bread can instead choose slowly-absorbed breads from Appendix III. If you're willing, try topping toast, a bagel or an English muffin with a teaspoon of olive oil before adding your favorite spread, and swallow 500 mgs of vitamin C. This converts rapidly-absorbed conventional bread and baked goods into more slowly-absorbed forms once in your system.

The next time you're in a restaurant such as Carrabba's or The Macaroni Grill, try dipping your bread into the olive oil provided. This helps make the bread less fattening, and adds antioxidant and vital oils. Also, if you must order fast food take-out sandwiches, have a banana or fast food salad first, and add a teaspoon of olive oil on the bread.

Pasta is another all-American favorite. The good news about pasta is that even if it's made with white flour, the glucose absorbs slowly, because pasta is recompressed. This makes it more difficult for our intestines to digest. Digestion will be further slowed if you cook it al dente, or enough to be firm but not soft, and avoid thin pastas such as angel-hair. When given a choice, select whole wheat, spinach or tomato pastas, because they contain more nutrients. If you're having white flour pasta at home, supplement some of the meal's nutritional deficiencies by having a salad first, and adding extra tomato sauce and a tablespoon of olive oil. If possible, do the same when dining out. If you can't tolerate gluten, quinoa pasta is a wheat-free alternative.

Chips are a big favorite among children of all ages. *BrightFoods* chips are made of stone ground whole wheat flour, with a touch of vital oils. Whether you make them using our pita bread recipe or commercially-available stone ground whole wheat pita, these chips are satisfying, and can enhance thinking ability.

Breakfast cereals are often made with enriched flour that's been stripped of nutrients. Processed vitamins are added and the end results are usually sources of rapidly- or moderately-absorbed glucose. So if you have to have breakfast cereal, instead of choosing one that may hurt your thinking and thicken your waistline, consider Kellogg's Complete or Zone Cereal. Eat it with either low-fat milk or chocolate milk, since they're both sources of slowly-absorbed glucose and many other nutrients. If low fat milk isn't appealing, try adding a slowly-absorbed fruit juice instead, or enjoy the cereal plain. Note: If you're a male over 40, you should avoid low-fat milk, as it may increase the risk of prostate disease.

In any case, start off with a piece of fruit, a drink of Tapple, or some vitamin C, since most breakfast cereals are relatively low in antioxidants. It also might be a good idea to eat some egg salad made with olive oil and spread on toast, since the cereals are low in smart proteins and vital oils, too.

Hot "instant" or "one-minute" breakfast cereals tend to be sources of rapidly-absorbed glucose. If you have a sweet tooth, you can add slowly-absorbed artificial or organic real maple syrup and a teaspoon of olive oil to old-fashioned oatmeal, with a hardboiled egg or a *BrightFoods* sausage patty on the side.

Potatoes have been in exile since the carbohydrate diet craze began. The basic assumption of these books is correct: Mashed potatoes are a source of rapidly-absorbed glucose. But this information may be misunderstood. It needs to be qualified: Mashed potatoes are a source of RA glucose when they're eaten on an empty stomach with nothing alongside them. To clarify this further, let's take an imaginarily visit to a lab where glucose absorption is measured.

Here, we determine a person's blood glucose level on an empty stomach. Then he eats a specific amount of potato, and his blood glucose level is checked shortly thereafter. Under these circumstances, the glucose in the mashed potatoes is absorbed rapidly. But because most people don't eat mashed potatoes solo, it may be unnecessary to ban the savory spuds. After all, they're a source of antioxidants and other nutrients.

There are two basic ways to reduce the glucose absorption rate of most rapidly- absorbed carbohydrates. As we've pointed out, one is to add olive oil to meals, and the other is to add an acidic food such as lemon, vinegar or tomato paste. So if we really want mashed potatoes, it's nice to know that merely adding olive oil transforms them into a more slowly-absorbed glucose source. Fresh "smashed" potatoes—that is, plain and cut into pieces but not mashed—are absorbed more slowly than fresh mashed with no other ingredients, because they require more intestinal digestion. Potato salad absorbs at a slower rate when vinegar is added. And as we've pointed out, other ingredients in the meal can bring the overall absorption rate down. *BrightFoods* smashed potatoes are absorbed even more slowly and are higher in antioxidants and fiber (see recipe in Chapter Nine).

Soda sales stand as testimony to America's love affair with sugar. Besides the beverages serving as a focal point of our latest carbohydrate witch hunt, soda is thought to be one of the many key factors behind the all-time high incidences of obesity and diabetes in this country among both adults and kids. Perhaps this is one reason that some schools have removed soda from their vending machines, many are considering it, and most will probably be forced to by legislation at some point. In addition, soda consumption indirectly depletes kids' bones of calcium—they usually skip milk when they drink it—and contribute to adult osteoporosis. No doubt soda adds to glucose surges and brown-outs, too.

"Sports drinks" are becoming increasingly popular as alternatives to soda, according to the schools we surveyed. But are our children professional athletes who require large amounts of glucose and salt due to their rigorous all-day workouts? If our kids don't get serious daily exercise, the sports drinks they chug may give them glucose surges, brown-outs, and salt accumulation. Researchers report that certain sports drinks absorb glucose even faster than soda!

This is one reason why the regular consumption of sports drinks in sedentary individuals can contribute to obesity, diabetes, and impaired thinking. Water, Tapple or slowly absorbed drinks listed in Appendix III are preferable to soda or sports drinks, because they're much less likely to create glucose swings and interfere with thinking.

A Brighter Ride:

What did the Cheerio say to the Complete flake?
Answer: I'll race ya!

Chapter Summary

- Brain cells rely on a steady flow of glucose in order to provide the energy they need for thinking, learning, planning, problem-solving, and feeling good.
- Rapidly-absorbed glucose can cause power surges that influence thinking and performance.
- Surges are usually followed by low glucose or brown-outs that can compromise energy, learning, memory, mood, and performance.
- Rapidly-absorbed carbs can cause fluctuations in glucose levels, making them function in the body like addictive foods that we repeatedly choose to eat in large quantities. Addictive carbs can contribute to thinking impairment, obesity, and diabetes.
- When eaten in the presence of the other medicinal food groups, a diet rich in slowly-absorbed glucose is more likely to improve thinking ability and a sense of well-being, as well as help to fight diabetes, overweight, and obesity, than diets heavy in moderately- and slowly-absorbed glucose.

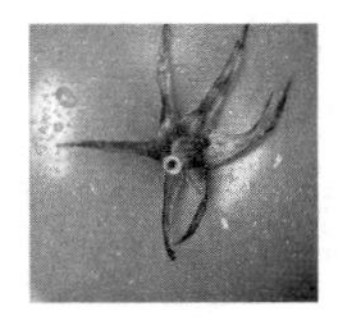

CHAPTER SEVEN
Toxins: Part of a Modern Diet

A surprising number of toxins enter our food supply. The list is long, and includes additives such as glutamate, preservatives such as nitrates, nitrites, and sulfites, non-nutritive sweeteners, salt, antibiotics, chemicals found in the water supply, hormones and pesticide residue. There's no cause for alarm, though, and we'll tell you why.

First, though, we should mention that our intention isn't to ruffle the feathers of health associations and food manufacturers. Instead, we want to work in tandem with them to provide a higher level of health consciousness among consumers, and to develop a clearer, more comprehensive master food plan that might improve individuals' thinking abilities and overall health.

With that goal in mind, we can share some facts with you. Food additives are chemical concoctions that substitute for nutrients our bodies need. They're ever-present in processed foods to stabilize them and make them taste "better" than home-made. Common table salt and some other seasonings found in nature are used in excess to enhance taste and preserve food. We find these and other additives in our foods, along with chemicals and toxins in the environment.

That makes today's food very different from that of our ancestors. Even water, which we consume daily either straight up or as the major ingredient in beverages, contains additives and toxins.

Brighter Water for Cooking and Drinking

We all know the taste shock associated with our first glass of tap water in a strange town. Even baked goods can taste different from region to region because of this variability. Water can also influence the flavor of beverages; it was reported that Christina Onassis often diverted her jet's France-to-South America shuttle to purchase cases of Coca Cola in New York. Drip coffee made with water from unfamiliar regions can taste horrid to us, and if we're accustomed to drinking tea or coffee made with filtered water, we can tell by taste which establishments use tap water.

But there's much more to water than just flavor: Proper hydration is vital to normal thinking. Drinking adequate amounts of water improves attention, learning, memory, and mood, while dehydration leads to fatigue, inattentiveness, mind-fog, and dizziness. But water hangs out with the strangest company sometimes. This is because, as physicists tell us, matter can't be destroyed, and the medicines we've taken and toxins we've dumped into the environment over the centuries linger there over time. Let's go fishing to see how our ecosystem responds to prescription medicines that have already passed through people's systems.

Millions of people—roughly one in ten Americans—have taken antidepressants such as Prozac and Zoloft. These medicines find their way into our environment to an extent great enough for fish living near municipal wastewater treatment plants to have detectable amounts of them in their body parts! And don't think the fish hiding out up in the Yukon are off the hook pollution-wise. They may be much less "happy" than their counterparts in the lower 48, because acid rain leeches mercury—a brain and kidney cell toxin, and depressant—out of the environment and into the crisp clean waters all over the world.

Therefore, we can assume that water that's used for cooking and drinking, including bottled water, contains tiny amounts of contaminants; a partial list of the ones found in drinking and bottled water that don't necessarily pose a health risk, according to the Environmental Protection Agency, can be found in Appendix IV.

Even a tiny dose of contaminants and toxins is undesirable, because an accumulation of toxins over time theoretically can affect your thinking and mood. Because we believe it's better to be safe than uninformed, *BrightFoods* recommends that at least one kitchen sink in your home have a water canister filter installed by a plumber; you can also buy a "screw-on" filter such as those made by Brita or PUR, which are convenient and affordable. It's easy to install, and fastens directly to most faucet openings. Costly "whole house" and "reverse osmosis" units aren't necessary. Filtered water is a flavorful and smart alternative to tap water, and saves money on bottled water.

Besides water, we often consume salt in abundance on a daily basis.

The "Salt Addiction" Theory

Salt is probably the most commonly-used preservative and flavor enhancer. It also appears to have addictive properties, because people who prefer heavily-salted food have difficulty eating their meals unless they're prepared this way, even if they know their habit is unhealthy. This on-going taste for salt and self-defeating behavior is sometimes a symptom of salt cravings, and may be part of the reason we love to eat fries or chips. We inevitably surrender to the lascivious salt craving, so we stop what we're doing, walk down the hall to the vending machines, buy a bag and enjoy those crunchy morsels. Then we wash our hands, get a drink of water and go back to work. And repeat.

In some ways, salt behaves like the addictive drug cocaine, which typically is used up rapidly. Once we get started with a salty snack or meal, we're often amazed at how fast it, too, is consumed. Salt seems to act as a food consumption accelerant. I call it "amnesic eating," because the chips or meals are gone before we know it, and our recollection is scanty. But uncomfortable bloating stands testimony to our deed. Perhaps an over-abundance of salt is the culprit when we find ourselves stuffed after eating our appetizer and salad, and wonder what we were thinking when the huge entrée we ordered arrives at our table. Before we can say "I ordered too much food," however, it's gone, and the dessert tray is beginning to look really good.

Then there's the opposite scenario: craving a drink to relieve the "salt-attack" brought about by an overdose. We're not exactly at the height of our game in terms of the ability to think straight in either instance. Our focus and ambition are reduced to relieving one of the two emotional discomforts at hand—salt-craving or salt-attack.

I have clinical experience with all forms of addiction, and I've believed for a long time that salt craving involves chemical instant messengers in the brain (recall how they tell us how to feel). It does appear that too little or too much salt alters attention, learning, memory, mood, and performance. In any event, research indicates that the right amount of salt stabilizes the ability to think. Some studies have shown that stress can lead to an increased appetite for salt, and that eating enough will then soothe the rattled soul. But as we've mentioned, excessive salt intake, with its associated water retention, is believed to disrupt clear thinking.

How might innocent table salt affect the brain like some prescription medicines and illegal drugs? There is strong evidence to suggest that salt and salt appetite affects not only dopamine in the kidney, but also "feel good" instant messengers, including dopamine, norepinephrine, GABA, acetylcholine, and opiates inside the brain. This might explain, in-part, why salty fries and chips have addictive drug-like properties.

In summary, the theory holds that when used in small to moderate amounts, salt is not habit-forming, and is beneficial to focus, thinking and behavior. However, when used in excess, salt not only compromises the cardiovascular system, but also makes us eat faster, gain weight, and think less clearly. So the next time you crave something salty and crack open a bag of chips, consider whether your sense of relief has something to do with a whole lot of "feel-good" messages going on.

Although you're likely to temporarily experience more feel-good instant messengers after eating foods containing salt or rapidly-absorbed glucose, when you consume artificial sweeteners, the good feelings probably go on break.

Non-Nutritive Sugars

Cyclamate and Saccharin were the forerunners to today's artificial, non-nutritive and low-energy sweeteners. You might find saccharin in some unlikely places; for example, it appears in some pharmaceutical products in small amounts as a sweetening agent. Little is known about the possible effects the two have on the brain or thought processes. Saccharin in infant milk formula has been associated with neurological changes in babies, including irritability and insomnia that lasts up to a day and a half. Similar nerve problems and headaches have been observed in adults, too.

There is considerably more evidence linking high-dose saccharin to problems outside the brain, including bladder cancer, diarrhea, eczema, increased heart rate, light sensitivity, nausea, skin reactions, sulfa allergies, tongue blisters, and wheezing.

Aspartame arrived shortly after cyclamate and saccharin, touting a low cancer risk. This all-inclusive safety "smoke-screen"—that aspartame is fine just because it isn't linked to cancer—is reminiscent of this warning from a seventh-century abbott: "Look for lion paws at the bottom of every curtain." So in the spirit of the good monk, we won't debate whether aspartame causes cancer, but we will look for signs of brain health risk beyond aspartame's "non-carcinogenic" banner.

This can be risky business, since history has shown that those who question assurances of safety, researchers and the "laity" alike, are ridiculed as being "caught up in an emotional issue." In this case, questioning the safety of aspartame may be more of a "defensive issue" than an emotional one. Whatever the motive, it's important for us to have as much information as possible regarding this widely-used and essentially untested chemical, so that we can decide for ourselves how safe aspartame is for our families.

Let's begin outside the brain, with no allusions to cancer. Aspartame is present in beverages and foods in the "diabetic" section of food stores. Although there may not be an explicit manufacturer's claim, diabetic consumers assume that it's safe. But there's no proof that aspartame-containing products help stabilize blood levels in diabetics, or are safe for them. However, it is well known that *diabetics need slowly-absorbed carbohydrates* in order for their brains and bodies to function normally. In my opinion, when diabetics stick to the slowly-absorbed glucose script and avoid high fructose syrup that also raises cholesterol, there's no place in their diets for non-nutritive sugar, because they're filling up on foods that contain the nutrients they need, rather than sweet-tasting, empty calories.

Also, we don't know how aspartame affects diseases besides diabetes. Some research has linked aspartame to nausea, dizziness, an altered immune response and growth hormone levels, pain perception, blood thinning and allergic reactions. But none of these studies used large populations, were designed well or were replicated. Therefore, we should assume that they're anecdotal, or founded on weak evidence. The following is based on a true story:

> *Jenna had been in treatment for poor impulse control, panic attacks, racing thoughts, and hyperactivity since the age of ten. By the age of 20, following many years of therapy, medication trials, and nutritional and exercise counseling, she was symptom-free for the first time in her life.*

After enjoying months of emotional stability, she inadvertently drank some "diabetic fruit juice" at her aunt's house. Within an hour, she experienced panic attacks, racing thoughts, and couldn't sit still. Her doctor made the connection between Jenna's behavior and the non-nutritive sweeteners that are sometimes added to Auntie's juice, flavored yogurt, gelatin, and gum. This taught her to be more careful about what she ate and drank. After Jenna made a concerted effort to avoid artificial sweeteners again, her problematic symptoms dissipated quickly, and she remained symptom-free for weeks.

She couldn't believe that one glass of juice could have caused so many emotional problems, so her doctor recommended that she drink a full glass of "diet" or "diabetic" beverage. She followed his directions, and the symptoms returned. Jenna has since stopped drinking artificially-sweetened beverages and foods, and lives a more happy and fulfilling life.

I've seen hundreds of my own patients, and heard about many others, who stopped using aspartame, and when they started again reported symptoms of depression, manic episodes, memory impairment, mood changes, nervousness, panic attacks, and temper outbursts. Only when they stopped taking aspartame did the symptoms subside. Although this doesn't prove conclusively that aspartame alters the ability to think, it does highlight the need for well-designed studies of how the chemical affects brain cells in people of all ages. These studies should be done by independent labs that aren't funded by special interest groups. Only then will we know whether or not aspartame affects brain function.

Another pitfall of consuming aspartame is that it's easier to convince ourselves that we're going to lose weight. After all, aspartame is added to beverages and foods labeled "diet," a word consumers usually associate with "weight loss" even if manufacturers don't use those specific words. But there's no proof that aspartame helps people lose weight. In fact, the reverse may be true. This applies especially to people who drink a product containing aspartame without eating during the day, and develop a serotonin deficiency that can stimulate cravings for rapidly-absorbed carbohydrates.

Serotonin is a feel-good messenger, and some people who drink coffee or other beverages that are sweetened exclusively with aspartame all day may be grumpy because they're experiencing brain shortages. We're to get out of the way of these people heading home on the interstate at five so they can binge all night on rapidly-absorbed carbohydrates, addictive fats, and salt.

Independent labs also need to conduct studies evaluating the connection between aspartame and weight management. Until then, the "diet" label may be deceptive to consumers.

Weight loss aside, it could be an aspartame-related serotonin deficiency that plays a role in the anxiety, depression, impaired memory, lack of drive and ambition, and learning impairment I've observed in steady consumers. Also, when used throughout the day without food, aspartame may indirectly deprive us of the slowly-absorbed glucose that produces energy and enhances thought. By dinner, levels of serotonin and glucose are down in Davy Jones' locker, while carbohydrate cravings are on a Sinai-high peak. Like zombies, all we can think is, "I want food!!!" This leads to evening binge-eating, mood swings from rapidly-absorbed glucose, and bloating, which can make us cranky to our loved ones, then guilty and disgusted with ourselves. This underscores the need for studies done under fasting conditions to evaluate the effect, if any, of aspartame on serotonin levels.

What about a little aspartame with a big breakfast, and later with a double-burger and large fries? There hasn't been any research done on adults or kids to see how aspartate, which comes from aspartame whether it's eaten with or without food, affects brain cells or the thought process, though moderate amounts of aspartate from other sources have been shown to affect how adults learn and remember. High amounts of aspartate can damage brain cells and receptors by over-exciting them to brown-out proportions or even death, a process called excitotoxicity.

Also, no studies have been done to evaluate how, if at all, the phenylalanine that comes from aspartame affects an adult or a child's thinking ability, even though the phenylalanine that comes from other sources is known to alter it. The same is true of the methanol derived from aspartame, when it's widely accepted that methanol from other sources causes brain poisoning.

My guess is that, when used in moderate amounts in a balanced diet, the aspartate, phenylalanine, and methanol from aspartame probably don't contribute to brain cell damage or impaired thinking ability in adults who are not allergic. However, there are many reports of side effects involving the brain that also point towards a need for studies other than those already done on cancer risks. Aspartate, phenylalanine, and methanol each have been linked to headaches. Aspartame is known to trigger migraines in about 11 percent of sufferers, and excessive use has been tied to seizures as well.

This must be studied further. Until researchers take a close look at aspartame's potential effects, when taken with a balanced diet, on brain cells, instant messengers and thinking ability, we can't assume that aspartame is okay for academic ambitions, learning, memory, and overall thought processes, especially in children.

Sucralose, marketed as Splenda, also touts a "safe" profile because it doesn't cause cancer or dental caries. Again, no one knows what lurks behind this smoke screen, either. Sucralose has just one blemish on its record, but that's probably one of the advantages of being the newest low-energy non-nutritive sweetener on the block. A study found sucralose-induced DNA damage in the gastrointestinal organs of rats. This study in itself, it should be said, has no medical relevance to humans, and certainly doesn't make sucralose unsafe for consumption.

However, sucralose hasn't been tested outside of the realm of cancer and dental caries, or assessed in any way with regard to brain cell or psychological functioning. No one knows whether there is or isn't an association between sucralose and weight loss, learning, memory, performance, the brain, heart, pancreas or intestinal health. Regarding bioavailability, no one knows whether sucralose increases, decreases or has any effect whatsoever on prescription medicine absorption. By the way, the non-nutritive sweetener in the processed juice that Jenna's aunt drank was Splenda.

Because low-energy sweeteners have only been deemed non-carcinogenic and okay for healthy teeth, *BrightFoods* cannot follow the position taken by the American Dietetic Association in 2004 and give them our blessing. It's our position that because non-nutritive sugars are low-energy, chemical concoctions that substitute for vital slowly-absorbed glucose; haven't been brain-tested or linked to weight reduction; have no antioxidant properties;

and aren't slowly-absorbed glucose forms, smart protein sources or vital oils, they have no place in a healthful diet.

One thing is certain: The emergence of sugar substitutes has paralleled the biggest surge in overweight and obesity in human history.

Glutamate

Substances such as aspartate, when present in large amounts, can increase the electrical activity in brain cells to the point of brown-out or destruction, a phenomenon, as we've mentioned, called excitotoxicity. The most common excitotoxin in food is glutamate, though it's thought to alleviate anxiety when present in moderate amounts. Perhaps being "addicted" to cheese, chips and similar snacks indicates a potential deficiency in glutamate and a need for a quick-fix response to the brain's difficulty in calming down under stressful circumstances.

Could it be that in addition to high salt, it's the high glutamate content of many snacks and processed foods that makes some people eat entire bags and boxes of goodies before they know it? Initially, eating glutamate can feel soothing, but when it's present in excess amounts, consumption can bring on a glutamate overdose, free radical formation, brain cell toxicity, and thinking impairment. The best way to avoid glutamate overload is to skip foods containing large amounts of it, because we know how hard it is to stop once we get started, how we can't have just a little, and how we're going to feel afterwards.

Veronica called her youngest son's doctor on his emergency phone late one evening in a panic. The doctor could hear items breaking and fists pounding flesh in the background as he was trying to gather information about his young patient. "No, it's not Jason! It's my husband and oldest son!" exclaimed Veronica, adding that they had never fought like this before. The doctor started asking probing questions, and discovered that the only unusual thing about the evening was that the fighters had seriously overeaten at a local all-you-can-eat Asian buffet.

Coincidence? Probably not, since excess glutamate consumption has been linked to poor behavior and memory performance, fear and seizures. The good news is that antioxidants appear to offset the toxic effects of elevated glutamate levels. This is why we believe that tomato puree, a concentrated source of natural glutamate and the antioxidant lycopene, is a valuable medicinal food that's not toxic to brain cells and promotes clear thinking. This is in contrast to the unchecked glutamate found in high fructose syrup, which is made from corn. Eating a side or two of foods containing bioavailable antioxidants when enjoying brighter fish and taking vitamin C with that bag of chips also helps minimize glutamate-induced cell damage.

Besides tomatoes and corn, other sources of natural glutamate include broccoli, mushrooms, oysters, and peas. The relatively high glutamate content in fresh broccoli, corn, mushroom, and peas is probably offset by their antioxidant content. However, once processing begins, especially with cheese, corn, soy, and whey, glutamate can be freed up to unsafe levels. (Glutamate originating from unnatural sources such as some manufactured food seasonings also gets into our food.)

Between glutamate that's naturally generated during food-processing and MSG that's added, large amounts of the stuff may be present not only in dishes served at Asian eateries, but in meals served in other types of restaurants, and even our own homes in various forms of packaged goods, including:

- Bottled: marinades, mayonnaise, nutrition powders, salad dressings, seasonings
- Canned: broth, chips, nutrition drinks, sauce, and soups
- Bagged: chips, popcorn, seasoning, snacks, and powdered soup mixes
- Boxed: cake, chips, cookies, seasoning, snacks such as wheat squares and fish, some cold breakfast cereals, and energy, cereal and diet bars

"MSG" or "glutamate" may not always be named as ingredients, but it can be present if the list includes any of the following words or phrases: autolyzed, hydrolyzed or textured plant protein; bouillon; broth; calcium or sodium caseinate; carrageenan; cornstarch; corn syrup; enriched; flavoring; gelatin; glutamic acid; lecithin; maltodextrin; monopotassium glutamate; rice syrup; seasonings; spice; soy protein; stock; ultra-pasteurized; whey; or yeast extract.

We do love convenience foods, so it's healthier for our minds if we eat a few washed tomatoes, baby carrots or other bioavailable antioxidants before indulging in items that are heavily tainted with glutamate. Natives of some European countries are living proof of why this is a good idea: Though in our culture it might seem that they're wasting time by cooking meals from scratch and shunning convenience foods, they have a lower incidence of obesity and live longer than Americans. Viewed in this way, the more convenience foods we eat, the more time we kill!

Being proactive is healthier than living in a bubble of fear, and *BrightFoods* can show us how to recognize which foods are high in glutamate, and to counter the effects of toxins in the environment. We can do this by trying to keep the ratio of medicinal foods to addictive ones high, without becoming obsessive or perfectionists.

Pesticide Residue

Numerous kinds of pesticides are used in agriculture to increase the quantity, quality and appearance of our grains and produce. Pesticides coming from sources other than food that's been sprayed contribute to free radical formation, oxidative stress, and cancer. While the American Cancer Society has suggested that there's not enough evidence to associate pesticide residue in food with breast cancer, even less is known about the connection between pesticide residue and other types of cancer.

We do know that certain types of pesticide residue from foods have been linked to brain cell damage and impaired thinking. When adults consume enough bioavailable antioxidants, however, they tend to counteract any negative effects the pesticide residue in foods has on thinking ability. This might not be the case with kids, who can take in a disproportionate amount due to their smaller size, and exceed the estimated daily limit established by federal agencies. Concerned parents may want to piggyback the kids' meals believed to be high in pesticide residue with antioxidants. This may not only help reduce the cancer risk, but also help them to think clearly.

Pesticides threaten both our health and the environment. Measurable amounts have been detected in wildlife and breast milk throughout the world. Pesticide residue can also be found in baked goods, dairy products, fruit, meat, poultry, and vegetables. Some pesticides can be found in higher concentrations in the fat portion of foods, but they also permeate non-fat portions. Where they're found and at what level depends on the type of food, what part is being examined, and in the case of produce, whether it's canned, frozen or fresh, as well as the length of time between spraying and harvest.

Let's look at three specific examples: tomato sauce, and strawberry and maple syrups. Washing and peeling is believed to remove essentially all pesticide residues from tomatoes grown in the US before processing them into puree or catsup. In contrast, pesticide residue in conventional strawberries is thought to be much higher than in tomatoes, even after washing. Perhaps strawberries, which are also high in antioxidants, off-set any brain cell damage that might have otherwise occurred from pesticide residue. Because no one knows for certain, *BrightFoods* recommends that adults, and especially kids, eat organic strawberries whenever possible, and if that's not possible, they should try to take vitamin C with conventional strawberries until they're proven to be safe.

With respect to maple syrup, in carefully checking each ingredient in Chapter Nine's recipes and in the *BrightFoods Cookbook*, we made some surprising findings. It turns out that we can only recommend organic or artificial maple syrup in our trademark breads and baked goods. Why? Although we love the people of the great state of Vermont and our Canadian friends to the north, some evidence seems to indicate that conventional pure maple syrup may contain formaldehyde. We don't believe formaldehyde levels are within the toxic ranges established for pesticide residue, and we're not saying that conventional maple syrup is unsafe. We're just saying that it's not an issue with the other two slowly-absorbed glucose forms.

Based on these three brief examples, it's easy to see how much variety there is in the levels of pesticide reside in foods and supplements. But there's much more we don't know about pesticide residue and their effects on thinking, and on disease in general.

Farm Animals on Hormones and Antibiotics

To increase milk production for commercial use, hormones are either injected into cows or mixed with their feed. Since there are no set standards regarding acceptable levels of these hormones in commercial dairy products, and we don't know exactly how much hormone spills into the milk we drink, we err on the side of caution. This is especially true with respect to children, because when these hormones come from sources besides milk, they're known to affect thinking ability and some organ systems.

For this reason, *BrightFoods* recommends organic low fat or fat free milk, and organic plain yogurt mixed with fresh fruit for children and young adults. Remember that low fat organic chocolate milk contains slowly absorbed-glucose, and is child friendly; young adults can enjoy it with a shot of espresso. If organic milk is unavailable or too expensive, conventional milk can still be beneficial to your health and relatively safe to drink.

In either case, calcium from other sources besides dairy and supplements, such as the foods listed in Table 7, might be wiser choices for people over the age of 40, who often require more calcium to ward off osteoporosis. We say this because billions of people worldwide don't get their calcium from dairy products, yet still have strong bones, while Americans who eat large amounts of dairy aren't less likely to develop osteoporosis.

TABLE 7 – Reliable Non-Dairy Sources of Calcium

Acorn Squash	Butternut Squash	Legumes	Turnip Greens
Almonds	Carob	Okra	Walnuts
Brighter Fish	Dried Figs	Oatmeal	Watercress
Broccoli	Kale	Sesame Seeds	

Sex hormones and other hormones are also given to farm animals because they have been proven to increase their protein mass with a minimal amount of feed. These hormones settle in the meats and eggs we eat, but because the Joint Food and Agriculture Organization/World Health Organization (FAO/WHO) determined 18 years ago that xenobiotic (unknown) residue in treated animal meat is safe, many feel that the issue's been put to rest. But when these same hormones come from other sources, such as prescription medicines or illegal body-building "steroids," or are taken in greater amounts, they're known to affect thinking ability, the onset of puberty, cancers that are dependent on hormones to grow, and other aspects of the human brain and body. Some experts believe that the FAO/WHO's position on xenobiotic residues is based on inadequate scientific data.

In addition, the meaning of "safe," and the age groups for whom the residues are safe, wasn't specified. It's true that the little research we currently have on hormone residue in foods doesn't provide enough evidence to associate them with disease, or to prove that organic meats and eggs are healthier choices. At the same time, however, there is no proof that hormone residue in conventional meats and eggs are safe for the psychoneurological development of children or adults.

Besides hormones, antibiotics are added to conventional animal feed, and found in the meats we eat. The extent of antibiotic residue in meat hasn't been adequately studied, and there's some concern that antibiotic residue in meat may change bacteria into forms that aren't easily destroyed with medicine. Antibiotics found in the foods we eat may also disturb the intestines, reduce vitamin K production, and cause toxic and allergic reactions.

Since the regulations and scientific justifications for adding hormones and antibiotics seem outdated, we recommend organic or "free range" poultry, organic lean beef and meats, and eggs, especially for children, if available and affordable. At the same time, adults who choose to stay with conventional dairy and meats may be in no real danger—but again, no one knows for sure.

A Little Ditty about Nitrites and Sulfites

Nitrates and nitrites are used to prevent spoilage in processed foods, such as meat. The nitrates and nitrites that don't come from food have been linked to cancer formation, possibly because they can increase oxidative stress (when free radicals are released and cells weaken). These chemicals, which are found in green vegetables or added to bacon, canned meats, cold cuts, ham, and hot dogs, may cause brain-rust and alter thinking ability when present in large amounts. At present, though, there isn't enough evidence to make a clear connection.

Sulfites are preservatives added to packaged and processed foods such as alcoholic drinks, cheese, dried garlic, lunch meat, red wine, and sausage. There is some evidence associating sulfites with skin, lung, and intestinal changes for the worse, as well as impaired thinking.

On a brighter note, a certain type of sulfate that's found naturally in the body called DHEA-S actually does a lot of good. It increases brain cell energy and networking, performance, memory, and well-being, guards brain cells from corrosion and reduces anxiety. Although you can buy it in stores in its processed supplement form, we believe that a balanced diet consisting of bioavailable antioxidants, slowly-released glucose, smart proteins, and vital oils, and which is low in additives and toxins, is the best recipe for excellent thought processes.

Supplements

Supplements are processed nutrients that are isolated, mixed with inactive ingredients and put into pills, while in nature these nutrients are found mixed with many other unprocessed active ingredients that facilitate good health. How well you absorb vitamins and minerals often depends on the presence of "family members," or facilitating nutrients. When they're present, the particular nutrients are absorbed well, and if they're not, they're not absorbed as well.

For example, the vitamin E in an avocado is thought to be absorbed more efficiently when taken with slowly-absorbed carbohydrates, smart protein, vital oils, and antioxidants, compared to processed vitamin E in pill form. Just as generic prescription medicines can be absorbed differently from brand name ones (think of Karen, the woman who had the terrible reaction to generic Prozac), our bodies may absorb the nutrients in fresh food more efficiently than the same nutrients that have been isolated, processed, and remixed.

One more risk to taking nutrients in supplement form is that the dose could be too high, potentially causing disease. For example, high doses of beta carotene supplement may increase an individual's risk of contracting lung cancer.

Vitamins and minerals are lost to whitening, shaping, heating, and milling, and ingredients that are added to make the supplements work better in the body can be altered by processing and pasteurization. Vitamin C, folic acid and thiamin are sensitive to these processing methods, and the more most foods, vitamins, minerals, antioxidants, herbal and other supplements are heated and otherwise processed, the less effective they may be. Storing supplements over a long period and in temperatures and humidity levels not recommended on the packaging also affects how well the body can make use of them. (The antioxidant mineral selenium seems to be an exception.)

BrightFoods believes the universe has a better handle on the delivery of vitamins and minerals than engineers do. Take its tendency to hold back very high amounts of free radical-forming iron and potentially toxic amounts of zinc in legumes. Few supplement manufacturers are sophisticated enough to understand that the "more is better" concept is a potential recipe for disease. The "more is better" mentality has scientists unknowingly processing soy with enzymes so that the "rich iron and zinc" stores found in beans can become not only bioavailable, but possibly toxic.

In this respect, the nutrient overload is similar to how the supplement vitamin E is toxic to the heart when taken in doses over 400 IU. A better idea: adding olive oil to your food, so your body gets a balanced amount of bioavailable natural vitamin E. When we do this in conjunction with a balanced diet, as outlined in this book, there's no potential for heart toxicity, and vitamin E supplements are unnecessary.

It's becoming clearer that nutrients in whole foods are more healthful than the same nutrients in supplements. Cancer researchers who equate nutrients from food with the same nutrients in supplements haven't been able to establish a cause and effect relationship between consuming the nutrient and preventing cancer. On the other hand, the American Cancer Society recommends five or more servings of a variety of fruits and vegetables each day. This recommendation is based on a solid link between cancer prevention and produce, regular physical activity, and maintaining ideal weight. These recommendations can also improve learning, memory, mood, and performance.

To Be or Not to Be: Organic Eating

BrightFoods recommends eating organic foods if they're available and affordable. Why? Because beyond free radical formation, we simply don't know about the damage that may be caused in our brains and bodies by eating food produced by non-organic or conventional farming methods. And because in some instances, organic produce, grains, and olive oil can be higher in antioxidants and lower in toxins.

For example, organic produce that's been juiced is thought to be richer in bioavailable vitamins, minerals, and antioxidants. Organic meats are lower or free of added hormones, antibiotics, and glutamine-containing broth, and are increasingly making their debuts in many conventional grocery stores. Organic eggs, low fat milk and yogurt are also said to contain low levels of hormones. Organic wine and hot dogs are made with little or no additives.

Organic farming is a practice that's good for agriculture and the ecosystem. It doesn't use any genetically-engineered seeds or crops, sewage sludge, long-lasting pesticides, herbicides or fungicides. Farmers using organic livestock practices raise animals that are healthy and treated humanely. They're fed organically-grown feed, and have access to fresh air and the outdoors.

Organic farmers rotate crops instead of using fertilizer, which allows the land a season to gain its strength back between harvests. They don't practice massive irrigation, because it depletes the soil. This method produces bright red, fragrant tomatoes loaded with lycopene, rather than light orange, nutrient-deficient ones. Also, pasteurization can denature nutrients in conventional carton or bottled juice. In contrast, fresh-squeezed organic orange juice or produce from a juicer can be the optimal antioxidant brain fuel.

But *BrightFoods* recommends gradually introducing organic foods into your diet, rather than making a radical conversion to eating only organic foods, because it's easier on the family, and more likely to become an enduring part of a healthier lifestyle.

Today, more and more organic foods are available and finding their way into mainstream grocery stores, as well as organic grocery stores like Whole Foods Market, which are springing up across the country.

Chapter Summary

- It can't hurt our thinking ability to drink and cook with filtered water.
- It's healthier to keep processed foods and salt to a minimum, because excess salt is unhealthy, can affect thinking and can make foods more addictive.
- Fake sugar isn't nutritious, and hasn't been proven to promote weight loss or to be safe in diabetics. Its effects on the brain are unknown, though it's associated with reduced energy levels, and it doesn't appear to serve a healthful purpose.
- Glutamate is an instant messenger. When there's too much of it in foods, it may be addictive and alter thinking ability, while in moderate amounts, it can serve a medicinal purpose in the brain.

- The amount of pesticide residue varies from food to food, and can potentially harm thinking ability or cause illness.
- Little is known about the effects of added hormones in meat and dairy on pediatric brain development or general health.
- Nitrates, nitrites, and sulfites haven't been proven to be safe or unsafe for brain cells and thinking ability.
- If you're accustomed to taking vitamin and mineral supplements, you may instead want to rely on wholesome foods to foster good health and clear thinking.
- Organic eating may be ideal for clear thinking, but you can be healthy on a non-organic diet.
- If you want to off-set the negative effects of additives and other potential toxins, you can try adding fresh, bioavailable antioxidants to your diet.

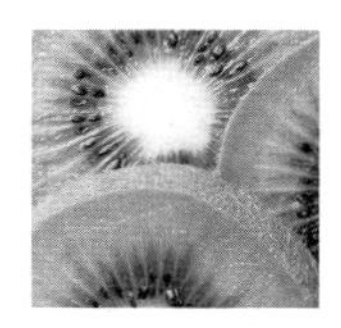

CHAPTER EIGHT
Immaterial Enrichment for the Brain and Mind

Woman and man do not live by burger alone.

If you want to think clearly in the long run, you need exercise, both physical and spiritual, as much as you need a balanced diet of antioxidants, vital oils, smart proteins, and slowly-absorbed glucose, with a minimum of additives and toxins. This chapter offers a smorgasbord of "immaterial" ways to nurture the mind, body, and spirit.

What do we mean when we say immaterial? We're talking about behaviors, rather than foods, which nourish brain cells and the mind, and are important to brain cell, intellectual, and emotional development. As with *BrightFoods*, immaterial enrichments such as sleep, exercise, meditation, prayer, karate, and yoga help learning, memory, mood, and performance by limbering up brain cell reorganization and networking.

Here's why these practices help. Enormous amounts of energy and information flow through more than 100-trillion synaptic connections within the brain and mind. Like inner city emergency rooms, police precincts, financial trading floors, and major news rooms, the brain/mind is a busy place relative to the rest of the body. In the pursuit of accomplishment and happiness, it constantly juggles thoughts—about the potential for reward vs. risk, self-preservation, knowledge, integrity, and judgment, to name just a few. Like the heart and lungs, the brain works automatically. Unlike those organs, however, it also has a "manual override." In other words, an individual can choose to undertake a lifestyle that reprograms brain cells for maximum efficiency.

Eating three *Bright* meals daily and *Bright*-snacking every two hours without incorporating at least two types of immaterial enrichment into your routine is a recipe for brain and body disharmony and inefficiency. Combining both food and good habits leads you on the path to a longer and more healthful life filled with both success and serenity.

Wake Up, Sleepy Head

The immaterial enrichment the brain loves to feast on most is an adequate night's sleep. Although we have the ability to learn while sleeping, we absorb much more information, experience, and strength when we're well-rested and wide awake. If we overdo it like modern-day Rip Van Winkles, we miss out on a lot of living, and feel increasingly unhappy and lost.

An estimated five million Americans sleep too much (hypersomnia), which is defined here as nine or more hours a night, plus naps. This can put the brain's hardware and thinking ability into a state of hibernation. Like bears stumbling about "drunk" on sleep while looking for snacks in mid-February, we have much less clarity, energy, and time to accomplish tasks that support well-being, academic achievement and an independent way of living. This cycle—hypersomnia, laziness, procrastination, lack of motivation and guilt—spirals downward, as feelings of unhappiness, low self-regard, inattentiveness, and fatigue grow stronger. Hypersomnia and all that it brings becomes an obstacle to learning, memory, mood, and performance.

What about too little sleep? Well over half of all young adults don't get enough sleep, and 40 million Americans suffer from insomnia. Sixty percent of the high school students we polled were tired throughout the day before participating in the *BrightFoods* lunch program, due to poor eating and sleeping habits. Sleep deprivation, along with conventional eating, can leave brain cells ravaged and exhausted. Insufficient sleep over prolonged periods of time prompts the mind to be less definitive and to "second-guess" itself.

Emotional and physical well-being is almost impossible under these conditions, and impaired focus, reasoning, creativity, and memory become the norm. We may also experience a motley buffet of emotions, consisting of anxiety, depression, frustration, impatience, intolerance, irritability, and worry. In addition to mind fog, our bodies sometimes remind us of how few hours we've been sleeping by giving us blossoming headaches, intestinal turmoil or neck stiffness.

There's a third sleeping pattern that brain cells aren't happy about, and that's binge sleeping. Binge sleepers stay up late on weekday nights and sleep in on weekends. Because we have century-old internal "sleep clocks" in our brains that have been pre-set by nature, fighting against them by binge sleeping can disturb brain cell plasticity and thinking, even in self-proclaimed night owls. Then there are people who regularly stay up for 24 hours or more, and then sleep for a day, believing that this will balance out their sleep "bank account." That's a hoot, when you take into account how they lose the time slot for brain cell resetting, errands, homework, and "honey do" lists.

In any case, correcting these pathological sleep patterns is often easier said than done, particularly when evening binges on foods containing glutamate or sugar substitute, sleep apnea or mood disorders are involved. In addition to chamomile tea, warm milk, or a hot relaxing bath, a sleep remedy for many people is 500 mgs of the amino acid L-tryptophan or 5 mgs of the antioxidant melatonin. (Note that users must have a doctor's approval first, since many supplements, even natural ones, can have side effects or interact with medical conditions or prescription medication.)

Though many problem sleepers turn to alcohol, this isn't a viable sleep-inducing option, because it converts in the body from a sedative to a stimulant within a couple of hours. A glass of wine taken at dinner can cause enough central nervous system stimulation by 11 pm to cause insomnia in many people, while a glass at 10 pm is likely to put some people to sleep by 11, but wake them up a few hours later.

When home remedies don't produce slumber satisfaction, it's best to turn to professionals for help. This is a good idea because sleep disturbances often signal the existence of another problem, and taking a prescription sleeping pill usually conceals it. Once corrected, sleepfests, sleep starvation, and binge sleeping, which can all alter brain cell and mind performance, happily become things of the past.

Where is the sleep/brain/mind nourishment connection? It's at the brain cell/mind level. Sleep disturbances decrease brain cell reorganization and hamper thinking, while a relatively fixed sleep schedule is believed to *promote* brain cell reorganization and networking, learning, memory, mood, and performance. Besides, getting on a regular sleep schedule puts many brain and mind functions in "neutral," allowing them to "reset" during sleep, just like our computers when we're not using them. Then we can begin the new day afresh, with optimal brain and mind performance.

It's vital to learning, memory, mood, and performance that we keep our brain cells alert and happy by sleeping about seven to nine hours, with lights out, around the same time each night. Shift workers—people who work through the night—aren't able to keep a sleep schedule close to our ancestral setting, which is around 9 pm through dawn. There are exceptions, of course; Thomas Edison possessed great thinking skills and only slept three to four hours per night. But this is impractical and unhealthy for most people. A good compromise might be to sleep regularly from around 11 pm until about 7 am.

Physical Exercise

Besides getting an adequate night's sleep, physical exercise can also improve learning, memory, mood, and performance, especially in someone who lives a relatively sedentary lifestyle. Increased physical activity enhances both plasticity in specific parts of the brain and in the organ overall with time, while sitting around leads to lessened cell networking. For example, the more we use our feet, the larger the part of the brain that deals with foot movement becomes. Also, to a lesser extent, the balance of the brain and mind increase in size.

In addition, regular exercise is known to quiet negative moods such as anxiety and depression, and to foster a sense of well-being. It's also been proven to help the heart, glucose tolerance, bone density, and possibly the immune system, while boosting brain-made "morphine," or endorphins, which further reduce stress and depression.

Most people don't exercise enough, and more than half of all adults don't exercise enough to avoid disease. More than 25 percent of adults don't engage in any form of exercise, and physicians advise about the same percentage of their overweight patients to increase physical activity. The problem is that most aren't able to put an exercise plan in motion for a number of reasons, including a lack of knowledge about the benefits, poor motivation, low energy, and insufficient direction or exercise counseling.

The first step in contemplating a personalized exercise program is plugging your weight and height into the Body Mass Index formula:

$$\frac{\text{Pounds}}{(\text{Inches})^2} \text{ or } \frac{\text{Kilograms}}{(\text{Meters})^2} \times 703 = \text{Body Mass Index or BMI}$$

19 – 25 = ideal weight

26 – 29 = overweight

30 – 39 = obese

40 – 50 = morbid obesity

BrightFoods doesn't recommend engaging in a regular exercise program, including walking for more than ten minutes per day, until either "overweight" or "ideal" weight has been reached. If you're someone who has an obese or morbidly obese loved one, it might help to understand this unlikely advice by imagining yourself holding a 25-pound dumbbell in each hand—50 pounds total—and going for a ten-minute walk. Chances are exhaustion would result after only a few minutes, and injuries could occur. How, then, are obese people expected to walk 20 to 30 minutes per day, a few days a week? Isn't this potentially too taxing to the cardiovascular system, bones, joints, discs, and body in general?

Regardless of weight, physician approval should be the next step in creating an exercise plan. This is especially true for people over 35 who have medical conditions that rule out a regular exercise program, such as uncontrolled heart disease and diabetes. With medical clearance, passive exercise can be built into the day's routine. For example, one good way to add walking to the day's events is to park far away from a destination. And staircases can be used instead of elevators, if they're well-lit and safe. If a building has an unreasonable number of floors, the elevator can be taken as far as two or three floors short of the desired destination.

The little gestures add up. Instead of yelling to get the attention of family members in other rooms, try walking over and knocking on their doors. Whenever appropriate, stand instead of sitting down, because it raises your metabolism. Squat instead of bending to pick things up, get a file from your cabinet or wash your car, and save your back while exercising. Take the garbage out during a TV commercial, or do a few push-ups while waiting for the shower to get warm. Not only is this physical exercise, but it gives the brain a shot of caffeine-like, stimulating oxygen, too. These are just some ideas. There are a lot of other ways to integrate physical exercise into your routine.

The next step is to find an active workout that suits your personality (in addition to some add-in exercises like the ones we just discussed). If it's practical, you can increase your motivation to get started by hiring a trainer. Also, no exercise routine will ever happen unless you figure out a good time to work it in, so you might carve out a 30-minute time slot, or one allowing you to burn off 300 calories and oxygenate your brain, that becomes part of your schedule four to five days per week.

When starting off, you don't have to be as gung-ho as a brain on dopamine. One or two days per week is good in the beginning, with a gradual increase to five days per week, always remembering that flexibility is important. Perfectionists and "do it right or don't do it at all" types often end up quitting. When you're behind schedule and only have 15 minutes to exercise, go for it. It's also important to view regular exercise as a means of living longer, so taking the time to exercise now potentially adds more time to work and spend with those we love later on.

The goal is to eventually get in 40 to 60 minutes of moderate exercise, burning off about 500 calories per day, five days a week, give or take a few minutes, calories or days. Reaching this goal faster or exercising for many hours isn't better, because it can unnecessarily accelerate your metabolism, leading to greater free radical formation. Just as eating a super-high-calorie meal produces larger amounts of these body pollutants that prompt disease, a marathon exercise session (burning over 700 calories) can be equally unhealthy because a disproportionate amount of disease-causing free radicals are also formed. Excessive exercise also increases the potential for injury and muscle aches that make you want to give up. Exercising in moderation makes you more efficient in your thinking when you conduct your daily activities, which can free up more time in which to relax.

For safety reasons, it's a good idea to do some stretching exercises before you begin. There are two types of activities: aerobic and anaerobic. Aerobic, or "cardio" workouts, include brisk walking, cycling, racquetball, running, skiing, stair climbing, swimming, tennis, and using the treadmill. Anaerobic, also known as resistance or weight-training exercise, requires some instruction in form and breathing techniques. Anaerobic exercises include bench presses, bicep curls, and push-ups. Some people incorporate both into their routines. Anaerobic exercise alone is not recommended if your goal is to become a better thinker.

Cognitive and Behavioral Therapy

Cognitive (related to thinking) and behavioral therapy involves learning ways to change the way you think and act, so that with ongoing practice, you can accept life on its own terms and maintain a predominantly positive emotional outlook. Everyone can benefit from therapy, including therapists. It can be especially beneficial when negative emotions control your existence.

If you've ever gotten into a fender bender with an angry, boisterous Neanderthal, it's easy to recall how other people's negative feelings can permeate your mind and being. Without therapeutic armor, negative emotions can be contagious. Fear and anger arising from other people's actions can flood your mind. Once inside, ill feelings and emotions muddle your ability to reason and make choices. Your body may react with raised blood pressure, headache, chest discomfort, muscle stiffness, intestinal discomfort or any combination of the above.

If you're frequently around stressful situations and abrasive people and have underdeveloped stress management skills, you can start to feel perpetually victimized, hostile, and that you're always treated unfairly. Under these circumstances, negative emotions dominate, even during peaceful stretches. It's easy to take on a defensive "I'm going to victimize before I'm victimized" stance. Such pessimists swear by Murphy's Law that what can go wrong, will. They may wear a smile in public, while feeling critical, negative, grumpy, and worried on the inside, except around people with whom they're very close.

Why not stay in a negative frame of mind? Like holding live burning charcoal, people harboring negative emotions do more harm to themselves, and run a higher risk of having anxiety disorders, attention deficit, impulse control problems, insomnia, obsessive compulsive behavior, temper outbursts, feeling unhappy, and assaulting others. And anger and other negative emotions are known risk factors for heart attack and other deadly diseases.

In sharp contrast, hanging around soothing people like the Dali lama, or a skilled and competent minister, monk, priest, rabbi or therapist can start shifting electro-chemical activity towards more positive emotions, and we begin to feel calmer and happier. Therapy can train us in ways of thinking and acting that promote feelings of serenity, and allow it to abide in us throughout the day. Before discussing one type of therapy, let's open a door to the mind, and take a look at the therapist's workbench.

The Therapist's Workplace

Because the mind is probably one of the most complex mazes we know of, getting a therapist to help us navigate through what sometimes is a minefield of predicaments may be just what the doctor ordered.

The mind is a wondrous work environment, and it's a privilege to listen to people and help them work through their most private quandaries. To appreciate just how amazing the mind is, let's imagine that it's structured like the US Department of Defense, with its main purpose being to preserve freedom and the pursuit of happiness. Think of the "upper," executive part of the brain as the Pentagon, which issues orders down the chain of command to the "lower brain," or the millions of employees, colonels and those reporting to them, who comply. From the executive brain's perspective, the lower brain, though vital to its operation, works pretty much behind the scenes and out of sight.

For us, this means that while we're actively pondering executive-type decisions, like whether to go to Mickey D's or The Cannoli Kitchen, there's a vast amount of intelligence, experience, and awareness that the upper brain isn't conscious of, but is there, nevertheless, ready to be used. Like soldiers or platoons who're called into action when needed, these concepts, experiences, images, and intelligence can be summoned in the flash of instant messengers from humongous memory data bases. Without actually thinking about it, the lower brain conducts extensive research about the pros and cons of each restaurant, such as the last time each was visited, and the general amount of wholesome food eaten since the last relapse. Before we can turn the car key, relevant data is sent up to the upper brain, and a choice of restaurant and often entrée is made without our consciously being aware of the reasoning behind the decisions. Granted, the choice can change within minutes or later, while we're standing in line, but you get the picture.

Now that we've inspected the troops, let's swipe our executive access card and go up top into the mind's Pentagon to see what the executive thinking committee is doing. Our first observation is that the upper brain is busier than the lower. As in the Pentagon, the workers are so busy and focused that we feel invisible. Enormous amounts of incoming timely information are sorted, sequenced, and prioritized here, seven days a week, including holidays. When stable emotions prevail, the VIP brain cells formulate solutions to problems, make decisions, and put plans in motion that yield the highest odds of reward, and the least exposure to risk.

Like the air force, army and navy, the brain has many executive thinking departments. Some muffle annoying, bothersome or distracting thoughts that would otherwise disturb the committee's decision-making capabilities; people with attention deficit disorder often find the muffling committee out to lunch.

Other committee members keep the executive board abreast of all the pleasurable rewards that could conceivably come out of a situation. The reward committee is almost always dreaming about romantic situations, acquiring more money or control, or engaging in leisure activities and otherwise pushing its own agenda, to the chagrin of the risk committee, which serves as the voice of reason. Because they each operate at different ends of the decision-making continuum, it's the executive committee's job to strike a balanced deal for each decision. When the executive board sways too far towards the reward committee, trouble often follows. When it moves off-center closer towards the risk committee, intimacy, making investments, and good times are less frequent.

We sometimes "hear" reward and risk committees bantering issues about in our mind like contrasting angels depicted in cartoons. A dialogue like this may sound familiar:

Reward Committee: No one appreciates me around here. I work my buns off so that others get rich! I'm going to march up to Scrooge's office and demand a raise, or I'll quit!

Risk Committee: You do that, and our sorry buns will be out of a job. Why don't you start scouting around for similar work, and compare what they're paying at other places to the total value we're currently receiving from Ms. Scrooge? And be sure to factor in base pay, growth potential, benefits, job security, and convenience.

Reward Committee: Yeah, sure! And when am I supposed to do all this poking around and calculations, smartass? They're working me to the bone around here.

Risk Committee: Stop what you're doing, and calm down. Take a deep breath in, and breathe out. Now listen. First, if we spent less time chattering in the hallways and playing golf on the computer, we'd feel less overwhelmed. Second, pick up the classifieds every morning on the way into work, and leave it in your trunk. Take just one hour each evening away from playing gladiator with Sara, watching those profound TV shows of yours and eating Chunky Monkey and Doritos, and look at the newspaper and Internet classifieds. Each evening, crunch some numbers. Now get back to work and be grateful you don't live in a cardboard box.

There are many other committees keeping a much lower profile, too. Mirror cells enable us to learn through observation—to mimic a dance instructor's steps, for example. Mirror cells also enable us to feel, for example, some of the pain after a loved one experiences a major loss.

This concludes our brief tour of the upper and lower brain. It's now easier to pursue the promised discussion on a type of therapy known as "positive imagery," which is a form of self-hypnosis training. Experience a few sessions with a skilled therapist and voila, the subject can bring about feelings of serenity on demand.

Here's how it works. After you assume a relaxing position and get yourself into a peaceful frame of mind, a therapist paints a pleasant image in your mind. For illustration purposes only (not recommended for home sampling), the therapist can ask you to close your eyes and imagine walking onto a deserted stretch of tropical beach. She might then softly and calmly suggest that you picture yourself lying in the white warm sand in a bathing suit, and gradually begin relaxing the muscles in your toes and feet.

Progressively, she'd recommend relaxing the muscles in your feet, calves, thighs, abdomen, fingers, arms, back, neck, and face. The therapist then might ask you to use your senses in imagining the light teal waves rhythmically curling to white on the sand and the light blue skies touching the horizon. You might be reminded about the sun warming your skin, muscles, and bones, and how relaxed you feel.

Focusing on the peaceful scene essentially allows all the other upper and lower brain chatter to cease, and you become more relaxed and calm. Though you appear to be asleep, the term "hypnosis," meaning "induced sleep," doesn't really describe what you've experienced; a better term might be "hyper-focused." Be that as it may, with additional training sessions and daily practice, you can learn to maintain a relaxed feeling throughout the day and evening, even when you're not in a hyper-focused state.

Therapists use this cognitive and behavioral method to help people with predominantly negative emotions "feed" the area of the brain involved in feeling positive emotions. Positive imagery and progressive muscle relaxation, a self-hyper-focusing technique, is one of many stress management skills therapists teach, and is the western equivalent of meditation.

Meditation and Prayer

Meditation and prayer can also be squeezed into our daily lives, and make for good immaterial "snacks." Both are forms of hyper-focusing, because when a dedicated practitioner pays attention to meditation or prayer, his mind is clear of distractions, and he develops or maintains inner peace. Scientific studies have linked these two practices with reduced aggression, anxiety, depression, pain perception, stress, suicidal thoughts, and violence. Both are also believed to strengthen brain networking and plasticity and therefore improve attention, thinking ability, creativity, learning, longevity, mood, self awareness, stress tolerance, and an overall sense of well-being.

Devoting a set amount of time each day for meditation or prayer, as well as practicing a shortened form of either during routine activities, isn't a new concept. In fact, it originated in ancient times, and predates stress management techniques learned in therapy by a couple of thousand years, as demonstrated by this old monastic tale:

> *A monk scurried to catch up with his stick-toting elder, who was just beginning his daily walk within their compound. The monk hesitantly asked, "Abba, is it okay to smoke while praying?" The abbott stopped in his tracks and curtly responded, "No." Then, as the elder resumed walking, he warmly added, "But it is okay to pray while you smoke."*

Two practices that are commonly observed by major religions because they're believed to enhance meditation, prayer or spiritual growth, are intermittent fasting and reducing caloric intake, as frequently as a day, a month or even half a year. In most religions, fasting and caloric restriction are voluntary. This is a good opportunity to talk about the effects of these practices on thinking ability.

Although researchers have shown that periodic fasting and caloric reduction can increase brain plasticity and clearer thinking, *BrightFoods* doesn't recommend these practices for purposes other than religious expression. Thousands of years of participation by the faithful have shown that intermittent fasting and caloric restriction are safe. In general, however, we should consume sufficient quantities of balanced *BrightFoods* calories daily to ward off hunger. The amount can vary depending on your lifestyle, age, and sex. If you don't get enough calories, you'll have a harder time feeling energetic and thinking clearly, while consuming too many makes you vulnerable to unnecessary free radical exposure, which can also impair thinking.

Adequate sleep, physical exercise, cognitive and behavioral therapy, meditation, and prayer are all associated with reduced anxiety and clearer thinking. Sleep aside, if these don't appeal to your personal taste, then read on.

When Cognitive and Physical Exercises Merge

Most people don't realize that they hyper-focus in order to relax. When you focus on an attractive person, news program or TV soap opera, your mind clears itself of thoughts and distractions, and you feel calmer. Reading and watching television can be relaxing, because focusing on a text or a program completely blocks out every woe in your mind within seconds. The resulting calmness is easily shattered by a loud noise, commercial or someone yelling "Have you heard a word I've said?" But can cognitive and physical exercise combine to make you even more relaxed and clear-headed?

There are absolutely no worries or preoccupations on the mind of a CEO and mother of three as she stands thigh-high in the breath-taking Penobscot River releasing fly line with a gentle forward and backward rhythmic motion. Not a care in the world invades her serenity as she focuses on placing the fly at the end of her line inside a one-square-foot pocket of water about 12 yards away. People skilled in pastimes from billiards to baseball and pursuits such as gardening and video games all hyper-focus in the same way.

The avid participant finds each of these activities relaxing. Hyper-focusing office workers can even find putting more hours in at work to be more relaxing than coming home to a chaotic household. The reverse may also be true. Let's look at more instances where exercise and hyper-focusing meld into one great state of well-being, beginning with an example that's thousands of years old.

Kung fu is more than just a series of dance forms, or "katas," patterned after the movements of animals such as the crane, praying mantis, snake or tiger. And it's much more than a series of combat principles. Kung fu involves the integration of martial arts with the tao, the philosophy of the ancient originators of these arts, as a way of life. Here is a thin slice of their philosophy:

> *A young student lying on the ground pondering by the monastery's lake asked his blind elder, who had just approached from behind, "Master, my parents have died and now I am gratefully here with many people, but why do I feel so alone?" The Shaolin priest instructed the student to close his eyes and tell him what he heard. The student did as instructed and said, "I hear the beetle. I hear the wind. I hear the tall grass. I hear the birds. I hear the dragonfly. I hear the fish." The priest chuckled and responded, "Why do you feel so alone in such a crowded place?" The sage then walked away, led by his tapping cane.*

In its purist form, kung fu entails a lifelong practice of both physical and mental discipline. For us, it can be a way to exercise both our bodies and our minds. If kung fu is not your cup of tea, perhaps one of its derivatives would serve you better. Kung fu is the mother of aikido, karate, and t'ai chi. When regularly practiced over extended periods of time, these forms can also exercise both the body and mind at the same time. These arts are also believed to increase brain reorganization and plasticity through both the regular kata (dance) exercises, and to cause an electro-chemical shift towards positive emotions in the brain.

Muscle-Stretching and the Mind

Muscle-stretching is also an exercise form that has been linked with improved mind function. Pilates, originating in the early twentieth century and a relatively new kid on the fitness block, involves smooth and steady muscle movements. It's a body-conditioning method thought to improve flexibility and tone, and to contribute to a leaner and longer physique. In addition to its use in healthy individuals, this potentially mind-nurturing wellness form is ideal for people suffering from arthritis or muscle weakness, when physician-approved and supervised by a trained instructor. You don't need expensive equipment to do Pilates, which can be done almost anywhere in as little as 15 minutes.

Yoga, which means "join," is a Hindu series of exercises intended to promote tranquility and insight, with heavier emphasis on the spiritual component than Pilates. It's an ancient practice that begins with a series of warm-up poses called "Sun Salutations." Once completed, the practitioner initiates the joining of mind, body, and soul through a system of controlled breathing, meditation, specific postures, and sounds. Yoga sessions can last more than an hour, but the improved body flexibility and overall sense of well-being that come with regular practice can be worth the extra time.

In addition to adequate sleep, one or more immaterial enrichments can make for a calmer body and a brighter mind. In the next chapter, we'll show how they work together with *BrightFoods* to provide the ultimate fuels for learning, memory, mood, and performance.

Chapter Summary

- Sleep disturbances are associated with impaired thinking ability, while getting about eight hours' sleep each night helps reset the brain, and increases brain cell plasticity, learning, memory, mood, and performance.
- Physical exercise improves regional and overall brain cell plasticity, mood, and thinking. It's best to begin exercising infrequently, and then gradually increase work-outs.
- Therapy can be an immaterial "food," shrinking activity in brain regions associated with negative emotions while stimulating brain cells associated with positive emotions.

- Hyper-focusing on a particular activity, person, place or thing such as reading, watching TV, or walking usually promotes a relaxed mind and body.
- Meditation and prayer are ancient forms of hyper-focusing that improve brain cell plasticity and clear thinking.
- Combining cognitive and physical exercises in the form of aikido, karate, kung fu, or t'ai chi can be beneficial to thinking ability.
- Muscle-stretching in the form of Pilates, or combining muscle-stretching with mind exercises, as in yoga, can improve thinking.
- Combining *BrightFoods* with immaterial "foods" can lead to optimal learning, memory, mood, and performance.

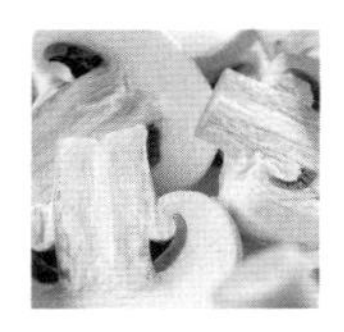

CHAPTER NINE

BrightFoods Sample Menus and Recipes

To recap: When we invest a little time lining up *Bright* meals and snacks for the next day, we potentially add years to our lives. Free radical formation constantly rusts brain cells and makes it harder for them to reorganize, network and maintain plasticity. Addictive foods weaken brain cells and thinking ability, while medicinal foods can improve plasticity, learning, memory, mood, and performance.

For optimal health, this means that we should get about 25 percent of our total calories from foods that are high in antioxidants and low in free radical-forming foods, such as smart proteins. And we need to limit our intake of not-so-smart proteins from whole dairy products and saturated fat-laden meats, even when they're organic, to less than five percent of our total calories.

As we've laid out in the preceding chapters, the best way to do this is to eat meals and mini snacks throughout the day that combine balanced amounts of bioavailable antioxidants, vital oils, smart proteins, slowly-absorbed glucose, and foods that are low in additives and toxins. *BrightFoods* combined with an adequate night's sleep and weekly exercise for the physique, mind and/or spirit can help develop and maintain optimal brain plasticity and clear thinking. The plan is also designed to help achieve and maintain ideal weight, and to decrease the risk for many forms of cancer.

A little *Bright* food goes a long way in delivering energy and shutting off appetite. For example, one slice of our pizza usually fills you up and helps you focus and feel energetic, and you're not hungry 45 minutes later.

The sample menus include a slight excess of beef, cheese, enriched flour, processed meats and foods to make it easier transitioning to the *BrightFoods* way of eating. The plan recommends a goal of eating one or less servings of each of the following per week: cheese, beef, and processed meat or soy. We also don't recommend processed vegetable oils and foods containing white, enriched or so-called "whole wheat" flour.

If you have a very active life style or want to gain weight, you can increase meal and snack portions. For weight loss, replace breakfast and lunch with a mini snack, and cut the mini snack portions in half.

Before sampling some *BrightFoods* menus, which integrate all the food groups discussed in this book, it's important to briefly address brighter eating for travelers and people who don't cook.

On the Run

People who are often on the run can gradually introduce *Bright* snacks into their diets every two or three hours. You can find some handy snack ideas in the slowly-absorbed glucose tables and the menus that follow. What we're about to discuss is far from ideal, but it's an improvement over how most Americans snack.

If caffeine is part of your team, it's a good idea to alternate a *Bright* mocha with each *Bright* tea; these can be made at home, school or work. If not, try low-sodium V8 with about a half-teaspoon of olive oil, Sixteen Carrot Jamba Juice, filtered water, or one of the juices from the slowly-absorbed glucose tables.

If breakfast cereals are part of your day's beginning, pick a slowly-absorbed glucose cereal and add low fat milk, chocolate milk, or unsweetened fruit juice. Top slowly-absorbed toast with a teaspoon of olive oil and then add a spread. For sandwiches, pick slowly-absorbed bread, and fill it with low sodium-and-additive delicatessen meats such as Boar's Head (bearing the American Heart Association flag). At Subway, you can order whole wheat bread with roast beef and/or turkey with lettuce, tomato, pepper, and olive oil. At McDonald's, eighty-six the fries and have the fruit and walnut or garden salad (easy on the dressing) before diving into a sandwich. Order thin crust pizza without extra cheese, and top with pepper and a teaspoon of olive oil where available.

For dinner, pick low sodium-and-preservative prepared dinners such as Lean Cuisine. Have a plum tomato or raw baby carrots while waiting for dinner to heat up, and add a tablespoon of olive oil to the meal. When ordering out, start with a garden salad, and ask for extra virgin olive oil and vinegar on the side. Request extra tomato sauce when ordering pasta al dente, and add pepper and olive oil. It's a good idea to *Bright*-snack into the evening to avoid binging.

Many more all-American and international meal and snack ideas appear in the forthcoming *BrightFoods Cookbook*. Let's look at four sample plans and their corresponding recipes, which follow the daily meals section below.

SAMPLE MENU 1 – Full Version

7:00 am	Tapple
7:15 am	Thirty minute thought-enhancing walk
8:00 am	*Bright* mocha (optional) or filtered water Sausage patty and tomato on a *BrightFoods* English muffin AM supplement (500 mg vitamin C or Ester C)
10:00 am	Tapple Unsalted walnuts (about 1/2 cup)
12:00	*Bright* mocha (optional) or filtered water Baby carrots, uncooked (about 1/2 cup) *BrightFoods* pizza 500 mg vitamin C
2:00 pm	Tapple Hardboiled egg
4:00 pm	Filtered water Banana
6:00 pm	Filtered water Field greens, cucumber and tomato salad with Yukari dressing Linguini and mini-burgers Corn PM supplement (500 mg vitamin C or Ester C) *BrightFoods* loaf of grain with apple (1 slice)
8:00 pm	Filtered water *BrightFoods* mounds of grain with oatmeal (3)
10:00 pm	Avocado (1/2) filled with shrimp and pepper
11:00 pm	Sweet dreams

SAMPLE MENU 2 – Full Version

7:00 am	Tapple
8:00 am	*Bright* mocha Plum Eggs or old fashioned oatmeal with maple syrup *BrightFoods* grain toast topped with olive oil & hummus, guacamole or peanut butter
10:00 am	Tapple *BrightFoods* grain muffin with banana
12:00	*Bright* mocha Veggie salad Poultry burger on a *Bright* bun Grapes
2:00 pm	Tapple *BrightFoods* mounds of grain with peanut butter
4:00 pm	Low-sodium V8 Pear
6:00 pm	Filtered water Tomato and cucumber salad Chicken tenders Asparagus Macaroni, broccoli, and cheese 500 mg vitamin C
7:30 pm	Thirty-minute thought-enhancing walk
8:00 pm	Filtered water *BrightFoods* grain bun with orange and cinnamon
10:00 pm	Peach and almonds
11:00 pm	Shut eye

SAMPLE MENU 3 – Full Version

7:00 am	Tapple
8:00 am	*Bright* mocha Mango salad *BrightFoods* chocolate pecan pancakes
10:00 am	Tapple *BrightFoods* mounds of grain with dark chocolate chips
12:00	*Bright* mocha Chips and guacamole Hot dog on a *BrightFoods* roll 500 mgs vitamin C
2:00 pm	Tapple *BrightFoods* grain bagel (1/2) with peanut butter and jelly
4:00 pm	Filtered water Dark chocolate (1/2 of a 1.5 oz bar)
4:45 pm	Thirty-minute thought-enhancing walk
6:00 pm	Filtered water Field greens and organic strawberry salad White chili con carne Wild rice, corn, and cashews
8:00 pm	Filtered water *BrightFoods* grain wedge with cocoa and peanut butter topping
10:00 pm	Chamomile tea Plain low-fat yogurt with fresh fruit and nuts
11:00 pm	Good night

SAMPLE MENU 4 – Short Version

7:00 am	Tapple
7:15 am	A few push-ups while waiting for the shower to warm-up
8:00 am	*Bright* mocha Slowly-absorbed toast with olive oil & spread
10:00 am	Tapple Unsalted dry roasted peanuts (1/2 cup)
12:00	*Bright* mocha Slowly-absorbed sub or wrap Orange 500 mg vitamin C
3:30 pm	Tapple Cherries (1 cup) M&M Almond or Peanut candies (1/2 cup)
6:00 pm	Red wine (1 glass) or filtered water Field greens salad Steak Smashed potatoes Raw baby carrots 500 mg vitamin C
8:30 pm	Thirty-minute thought-enhancing walk
9:00 pm	Kellogg's Complete with blueberries and skim milk (small bowl)
10:30 pm	Hot bath and chamomile tea
11:00 pm	Reset and re-plasticize brain cells

Corresponding Recipes and Trademark *BrightFoods* Baked Goods

Though not essential to *Bright* eating, all recipes were developed and tested by Dr. Cocores using organic ingredients.

Drink Up, Me Hardies!

Tapple (A, S, L)

Green, regular (black), white, or red tea steeped for about four minutes and poured over ice with two shot glasses-full of chilled unsweetened apple, mango or other slowly-absorbed fruit juice added.

For larger quantities, pour ten cups of filtered water into a drip coffee-maker reservoir. Put five tea bags inside the coffee pot with the tags hanging over the outside, close the top and replace the pot in the coffee-maker. Turn it on; after the pot is full of hot tea, allow steeping for about four minutes. Remove the tea bags.

REMINDERS: Decaffeinated and bottled teas may be antioxidant-depleted. Also, "decaffeinated" means "less caffeine," not "caffeine-free." Only excess caffeine is reportedly unhealthy. A surplus of antioxidants makes drinking conventional tea and apple juice worthwhile, despite possible trace amounts of toxins.

Bright Mocha (A, P, S, L)

This is for coffee lovers (people who don't drink coffee can replace it with tea, filtered water or a juice from the slowly-absorbed glucose tables). Add a 1/4 to 1/2 cup of warmed low fat chocolate milk to a mug containing coffee or a shot of espresso.

LEGEND
A = Antioxidant
O = Vital Oil
P = Smart Protein
S = Slowly-Absorbed Glucose
L = Lower in Additives or Toxins

BREAKFAST

Sausage Patty and Tomato Muffin (A, O, P, S, L)

1 *BrightFoods* English muffin – recipe in Bakery section

1 sausage patty, no preservatives or additives – recipes below

1 1/4 inch tomato slice

1 teaspoon extra virgin olive oil, filtered (here on referred to as "olive oil")

1 tablespoon catsup, guacamole, hummus or mustard

Lightly toast muffin and pour about a teaspoon of olive oil on one half. Spread catsup, guacamole, hummus, or mustard on the other half. Place patty and tomato in-between.

Sausage Patties

1 tablespoon ground mustard

1 teaspoon rubbed sage

1 teaspoon ground fennel seeds

1 teaspoon ground thyme

1/2 teaspoon white pepper

1/4 teaspoon sea salt

1 lb ground chicken or turkey

1 tablespoon olive oil

Preheat oven to 325 degrees. Add mustard, sage, fennel, thyme, pepper, and salt to a medium size bowl. Stir spices and spread them out over the bottom of the bowl. Add the meat and then flip it over. Knead until the spices are evenly distributed. Add oil and knead briefly. Use an egg fry ring as a mold on an oiled baking sheet (stainless steel bakeware preferred to avoid possible aluminum leaching). Tablespoon the meat into an egg ring forming a 3/8 inch thick patty. Repeat eight more times using the same ring. Spray the tops with olive oil using a mister. Bake the patties for 20 minutes. Flip, spray and bake for about 15 to 20 minutes or until well done.

Makes nine patties.

Can be frozen and reheated as needed.

See the end of Medical Journal Sources to find ingredients and utensils listed in this chapter.

Vegan Breakfast Patties

2 cups kidney beans, cooked

1 cup wild rice, cooked

1 tablespoon ground mustard

1 teaspoon rubbed sage

1 teaspoon ground fennel

1 teaspoon ground thyme

1 teaspoon black pepper

1/4 teaspoon sea salt

1/4 cup pectin, liquid

2 tablespoons olive oil

1/2 cup stone ground whole wheat flour

1/2 cup filtered water

Preheat oven to 350 degrees. Combine beans, rice, mustard, sage, fennel, thyme, pepper, salt, pectin, and oil. Stir together and smash, using a potato masher. Stir the flour and water together in a measuring cup. Thoroughly stir the flour into the bean mixture. Use an egg fry ring on an oiled baking sheet as a mold. Spoon the bean mixture into an egg ring forming a 3/8 inch thick patty. Repeat nine more times using the same ring. Spray the tops with olive oil. Cook for 15 minutes. Flip, spray, and bake for another 15 minutes.

Makes ten patties.

LEGEND
A = Antioxidant
O = Vital Oil
P = Smart Protein
S = Slowly-Absorbed Glucose
L = Lower in Additives or Toxins

Answers for vegan breakfast patties:

Kidney beans, cooked – A, O, P, S, L
Wild rice, cooked – A, P, S, L
Ground mustard – A, L
Rubbed sage – A, L
Ground fennel – A, L
Ground thyme – A, L
Black pepper – A, L
Sea salt – L
Pectin, liquid – A
Olive oil – A, O, L
Stone ground whole wheat flour – A, O, P, S, L
Filtered water – L

Plum, Eggs, and Toast (A, O, P, S, L)

A sliced plum or other slowly-absorbed fruit

Egg(s) prepared with olive oil or old fashioned oatmeal with organic maple syrup and olive oil

One slice *BrightFoods* grain bread or slowly-absorbed bread lightly toasted and topped with one teaspoon olive oil

BrightFoods Grain Bread (A, O, P, S, L)

1 3/4 cups warm filtered water

1/4 teaspoon raw sugar

2 pkgs dry yeast

5 cups stone ground whole wheat flour

1/2 teaspoon sea salt

1/2 cup olive oil

1/2 cup organic maple syrup

Pour water, sugar, and yeast into a container. Stir and allow to stand for ten minutes. Pour two cups of flour into a medium mixing bowl and stir in salt. Warm olive oil and maple syrup in a small sauce pan. Stir the yeast with the flour until dough is pasty. Stir in the oil and syrup. Combine with three cups of flour. Flour a counter area and knead for about eight minutes. Place the dough into a floured bread pan about 9x5x3 in size. Cover and let rise for about 40 minutes, or until double the size.

Bake in oven preheated to 350 degrees for about 60 minutes or until light brown, spraying with water every 15 minutes. Let cool, then use a butter knife to separate from all sides. Turn pan upside down and remove the loaf. After it cools down, cut the loaf into slices and refrigerate.

LEGEND
A = Antioxidant
O = Vital Oil
P = Smart Protein
S = Slowly-Absorbed Glucose
L = Lower in Additives or Toxins

BrightFoods Chocolate Pecan Pancakes (A, O, P, S, L)

2 cups stone ground whole wheat flour

1/4 cup pecans, finely chopped

1 1/2 tsps baking powder

3/4 teaspoon baking soda

1/4 teaspoon sea salt

3 cups low fat chocolate milk

3 eggs, separated

1/4 cup olive oil

2 tablespoons organic maple syrup

Combine flour, pecans, baking powder, baking soda, and salt in a medium size bowl; stir together. Add milk, egg yolks, olive oil, and maple syrup; stir together. Preheat oiled skillet over a medium flame. Beat egg whites until they stiffen, and fold into the batter. Scoop pancake batter onto the skillet using a ladle, and heat until light brown on each side—about four minutes on one side then three minutes on the other. Cool down skillet as needed with a little water, and lightly oil.

Makes 12 to 16 pancakes.

Can be refrigerated and reheated as needed.

Vegan Version

2 cups stone ground wheat flour

1/4 cup finely chopped pecans

4 tablespoons pectin powder, premium

1 1/2 tsps baking powder

3/4 teaspoon baking soda

1/4 teaspoon sea salt

3 1/2 cups chocolate almond or rice drink

1/4 cup olive oil

1/4 cup organic maple syrup

Combine dry ingredients and stir together. Preheat oiled skillet over a medium flame. Add wet ingredients to dry and whisk together. Scoop pancake batter onto the skillet using a ladle, and heat until light brown on each side—about three minutes on one side then two minutes on the other. Cool down skillet with a little water and lightly oil as needed. Whisk each time before scooping batter.

Makes 12 to 16 pancakes.

MINI SNACKS

Fresh Fruits and Vegetables (A, P, S, L) – Carefully washed fruits and vegetables

Fruit – Apples, bananas, cherries, figs, grapefruit, grapes, mangoes, oranges, peaches, pears, and plums

Vegetable – Artichokes, asparagus, avocadoes, broccoli, cabbages, carrots, cauliflower, celery, corn, cucumbers, eggplants, garlic, green beans, lettuce, mushrooms, peas, peppers, sweet potatoes, and zucchini

---

Veggie Salad (A, O, P, S, L)

1 cup diced celery

1 cup diced carrots

1 cup hummus, guacamole, or peanut butter mixed with filtered water (1:1)

LEGEND
A = Antioxidant
O = Vital Oil
P = Smart Protein
S = Slowly-Absorbed Glucose
L = Lower in Additives or Toxins

BrightFoods Loaf of Grain with Apple (A, O, P, S, L)

1 1/2 cups stone ground whole wheat flour

1/2 cup old fashioned oats

1/4 cup chopped walnuts

1/4 cup raw sugar

1 tablespoon baking powder

1 teaspoon cinnamon

1/2 teaspoon baking soda

1/4 teaspoon sea salt

3/4 cup mashed apple or applesauce

3/4 cup fat free milk or water

1/4 cup olive oil

1/4 cup organic maple syrup

1 egg or 2 tablespoons liquid pectin

Preheat oven to 375 degrees. In a medium size bowl, combine flour, oats, walnuts, sugar, baking powder, cinnamon, baking soda, and salt. Stir and make a large impression in the center with a tablespoon. Whisk the remaining ingredients together in a small bowl and pour into the impression. Mix until dry ingredients are moistened. Pour into oiled 5x9x2 pan. Bake on top rack 45 to 50 minutes, or until light brown.

For muffins, spoon batter into muffin pan about 2/3 full. Bake for about 25 minutes or until light brown. Allow to cool; separate from sides using a butter knife. Keep refrigerated.

Makes 12 muffins.

BrightFoods Mounds of Grain with Oatmeal (A, O, P, S, L)

1/2 cup olive oil

1/2 cup filtered water

3/4 cup organic maple syrup

1 egg or 3 tablespoons liquid pectin

1 teaspoon vanilla

3 cups old fashioned oats

1 cup stone ground whole wheat flour

1/2 cup chopped walnuts

1 teaspoon baking soda

1/4 teaspoon sea salt

Preheat oven to 350 degrees. Whisk olive oil, water, and maple syrup in a small bowl. Beat in egg and vanilla. In a separate bowl, stir together the dry ingredients. Combine the wet with the dry ingredients until uniformly moistened. Holding a tablespoon in each hand, cup dough in-between and push out almond shaped mounds about 1 inch apart onto baking sheets. Bake on the top oven rack one sheet at a time for 30 minutes, or until light brown. Keep refrigerated

Makes about 36 mounds.

LEGEND
A = Antioxidant
O = Vital Oil
P = Smart Protein
S = Slowly-Absorbed Glucose
L = Lower in Additives or Toxins

BrightFoods Grain Muffins with Banana (A, O, P, S, L)

1 1/2 cups stone ground whole wheat flour

1/2 cup old fashioned oats

1/4 cup chopped walnuts

1/4 cup raw sugar

1 tablespoon baking powder

1/2 teaspoon baking soda

1/2 teaspoon cinnamon or nutmeg

1/4 teaspoon sea salt

2 medium bananas mashed

1 egg or 3 tablespoons liquid pectin

3/4 cup fat free milk or water

1/4 cup organic maple syrup

1/4 cup olive oil

Preheat oven to 375 degrees. Combine flour, oats, walnuts, sugar, baking powder, baking soda, cinnamon, and salt in a mixing bowl. Make an impression in the center with a tablespoon. Combine remaining ingredients in a small bowl and mix thoroughly so that there are no clumps of banana. Add the wet ingredients to the dry ingredients and mix until they're moistened. Spoon into oiled muffin pans about 2/3 full. Bake 25 minutes or until light brown. Allow to cool and separate from sides using a butter knife. Keep refrigerated. Makes 12 muffins.

BrightFoods Mounds of Grain with Peanut Butter (A, O, P, S, L)

2/3 cup peanut butter, no sugar added

1/2 cup olive oil

1 cup filtered water

1/3 cup organic maple syrup

1 egg or 3 tablespoons liquid pectin

1/2 teaspoon vanilla

2 cups stone ground whole wheat flour

1 cup old fashioned oats

1/3 cup raw unsalted peanuts, chopped

1/2 teaspoon baking soda

1/4 teaspoon sea salt

Preheat oven to 350 degrees. Warm the peanut butter in a double boiler. Whisk the olive oil, water, maple syrup, egg, and vanilla together in a small bowl. Beat in the warm peanut butter. Combine the flour, oats, peanuts, baking soda, and salt in a separate bowl. Thoroughly moisten the dry ingredients with the wet. Holding a tablespoon in each hand, slide out rounded tablespoonful onto lightly oiled baking sheets about one inch apart. Bake each sheet one at time on the top rack for 20 to 25 minutes, or until light brown. Keep refrigerated.

Makes about 38 mounds.

LEGEND
A = Antioxidant
O = Vital Oil
P = Smart Protein
S = Slowly-Absorbed Glucose
L = Lower in Additives or Toxins

BrightFoods Mounds of Grain with Dark Chocolate Chips (A, O, P, S, L)

1/4 cup olive oil

1/4 cup organic maple syrup

1 cup filtered water

1 egg or three tablespoons liquid pectin

1 teaspoon vanilla

2 cups stone ground whole wheat flour

1 cup dark chocolate chips

1 cup chopped walnuts, peanuts, pecans, or sunflower seeds

1/2 cup old fashioned oats

1/4 cup raw sugar

1/2 teaspoon baking soda

Preheat oven to 350 degrees. Whisk together in a small bowl the oil, maple syrup, water, egg, and vanilla. In a separate medium size bowl stir together the remaining ingredients. Add the wet ingredients to the dry and stir until thoroughly moistened. Press batter in-between two tablespoons and push out rounded tablespoonfuls onto oiled baking sheets about one inch apart. Bake on top rack one sheet at a time for 20 to 25 minutes or until light brown. Keep refrigerated.

Makes about 36 mounds.

BrightFoods Grain Bagels

2 pkgs dry yeast

1 cup warm filtered water

4 tablespoons blueberry jam, organic strawberry jam or maple syrup

1/2 teaspoon sea salt

1/4 cup old fashioned oats

1/4 cup olive oil

2 1/2 cups stone ground whole wheat flour

2 quarts filtered water

In a large mixing bowl, dissolve yeast in warm water and stir in one cup of flour, jam or syrup, salt, and oats. Stir ingredients. Stir in the oil. Add the remaining 1 1/2 cups of flour. Knead on a floured surface for about eight minutes, or until smooth and elastic. Place in oiled bowl, then turn oiled side up, cover and let rise for about 30 minutes, or until double in size.

Flatten down the dough and divide into eight equal parts. Shape each part into a ball and punch a hole in the middle of each ball on a cutting board, using a short piece of 1/2 inch tubing. Allow bagels to rise for 40 minutes or until double the size.

Bring two quarts of water to a boil, reduce the heat, and add as many bagels as can float. Simmer four minutes on one side and three minutes on the other. Preheat oven to 375 degrees. Drain on towel and repeat with remaining bagels. Bake parboiled bagels on oiled baking sheet for 30 minutes or until light brown.

Makes eight bagels.

LEGEND
A = Antioxidant
O = Vital Oil
P = Smart Protein
S = Slowly-Absorbed Glucose
L = Lower in Additives or Toxins

BrightFoods Grain Wedges with Cocoa and Peanut Butter Topping (A, O, P, S, L)

1 1/4 cups stone ground whole wheat flour

1/4 cup raw sugar

1/4 cup cocoa

1 teaspoon baking powder

1/2 teaspoon baking soda

1/4 teaspoon sea salt

1 1/4 cup filtered water

1/4 cup olive oil

1/4 cup organic maple syrup

1/2 cup peanut butter, no sugar added

Stir flour, sugar, cocoa, baking powder, baking soda, and salt together. Wisk water, olive oil, and maple syrup, and stir into the dry ingredients. Pour into oiled eight-inch round pan and bake at 350 degrees for 50 to 60 minutes or until done. Top with peanut butter. Keep refrigerated.

Serves eight.

For muffins, spoon into lightly oiled muffin pan about 2/3 full and bake for about 25 minutes, or until done.

Makes 12 muffins.

BrightFoods Pizza (A, O, P, S, L)

Pizza Dough

1 cup warm filtered water

1/4 teaspoon raw sugar

1 pkg dry yeast

1/4 teaspoon sea salt

1/4 cup organic maple syrup

1/4 cup olive oil

3 cups stone ground whole wheat flour

Pour water, sugar, and yeast into a container. Stir and allow standing for five minutes. Pour one cup of flour into a medium bowl and stir in salt. Add warm water containing yeast into the flour and mix with a spoon until dough is pasty. Thoroughly stir in the syrup and oil. Add two cups of flour and collect into a dough ball. Knead on a firm surface for about five minutes. Flatten dough into a floured bowl. Lightly flour the top. Cover and let rise for about one hour or until double the size. Makes a 16" thin crust pizza.

LEGEND
A = Antioxidant
O = Vital Oil
P = Smart Protein
S = Slowly-Absorbed Glucose
L = Lower in Additives or Toxins

Pizza Sauce

1/4 cup olive oil

1 garlic clove pressed

6 ozs tomato paste

18 ozs filtered water

1 tablespoon mustard

1 teaspoon dried oregano

1 teaspoon celery flakes

1/2 teaspoon black pepper

1/4 teaspoon turmeric

Heat olive oil and garlic in a sauce pan until the garlic begins to sizzle. Then lightly sauté the tomato paste. Stir in water, and remaining ingredients. Bring to a boil, cover, and simmer on a low flame for an hour, stirring occasionally.

Cheese Topping (optional)

10 oz mozzarella cheese (no BGH-bovine growth hormone, part skim preferred)

1/2 cup shredded reduced fat sharp cheddar or 2 tablespoons grated Parmegiano

Preheat oven to 375 degrees. Smack dough to remove air bubbles. Roll out dough on a floured surface. Fit onto 17" lightly floured circular pan. Form a lip of dough around the edge. Top with pizza sauce. If cheese topping is used, spray with olive oil mister. Bake on lower oven rack for 15 to 20 minutes or until crust is light brown.

Poultry Burgers (A, O, P, S, L)

2 tablespoons olive oil

1 small onion finely chopped

1/2 cup stone ground whole wheat flour

1 tablespoon cilantro

1 tablespoon mustard, ground

1/4 teaspoon black pepper

1/4 teaspoon paprika

1/4 teaspoon sea salt

1/4 teaspoon turmeric

1 lb ground chicken or turkey

Preheat oven to 325 degrees. Sauté onions in a sauce pan containing olive oil and remove from flame. In a small bowl, add flour, cilantro, mustard, black pepper, paprika, sea salt, and turmeric, and mix. Combine the ground meat and cooled onions, and mix together by hand. Flatten the meat and sprinkle the spiced flour on top. Knead until spices are uniformly distributed. Cut the meat into five equal pieces. Shape into 1/2 inch thick burgers and place on a baking sheet. Bake on top oven rack for 20 minutes. Flip and bake for 15 to 20 minutes more, or until well done.

Makes 5 burgers.

Serve on *BrightFoods* burger buns – Recipe in the Bakery section.

LEGEND
A = Antioxidant
O = Vital Oil
P = Smart Protein
S = Slowly-Absorbed Glucose
L = Lower in Additives or Toxins

Vegan Burgers

Shape vegan spheres recipe found in the Dinner section into 1/2 inch thick burgers and bake as directed in that recipe.

Guacamole, Chips, and Hot Dogs (A, O, P, S, L)

Guacamole

2 avocados

1 small tomato, diced

1/4 cup hummus (optional)

1/4 cup cilantro finely chopped (or 1/8 cup dried)

1 tablespoon lime juice

1/2 teaspoon chili powder

1/4 teaspoon white pepper

1/4 teaspoon sea salt

Mash ingredients together until smooth.

Chips

Preheat oven to 350 degrees. Using a pizza cutter, cut five pita loaves made from stone ground whole wheat bread into eight slices. Separate each slice into two chips. Spread chips out on two cookie sheets and bake one sheet at a time for about 12 minutes. Remove from oven and allow chips to cool for about five minutes. Optional: Lightly spray with olive oil.

Hot Dogs

Low sodium and low nitrate beef franks with no artificial colors, flavors, antibiotics, steroids, pesticides, fillers or byproducts.

BrightFoods hot dog rolls (in the Bakery section) or Snuggles (see Internet Addresses after Medical Journal Sources).

Brighter Sandwiches

BrightFoods, German dark wheat, nine to 12 grain, sourdough, or pumpernickel sub roll or wrap

Spread hummus or guacamole and fill the slowly-absorbed roll or wrap with chicken tenders or mini-burgers, field greens, and tomato, and sprinkle with olive oil. Add pepper and lightly salt.

LEGEND
A = Antioxidant
O = Vital Oil
P = Smart Protein
S = Slowly-Absorbed Glucose
L = Lower in Additives or Toxins

DINNER

Field Greens, Cucumber, and Tomato Salad (A, O, P, S, L)

Yukari Dressing

1 Fuji apple

2 small carrots

1/4 cup ginger

4 tablespoons olive oil

2 tablespoons rice vinegar

1/2 teaspoon sea salt

Juice apple, carrots, and ginger, and add the remaining ingredients. Place field greens and 3/4 of Yukari dressing into a large plastic bag, seal, and shake. Empty the contents into a large bowl. Add cut tomato and cucumber and the rest of the dressing to the bag, seal it, and do the Watusi. Pour the contents atop the greens. Refrigeration and reuse of Yukari dressing is not recommended.

—OR—

Oil and Vinegar Dressing

First toss field greens, tomato, and cucumber in balsamic vinegar. Then add pepper, lightly salt and toss. Lastly, add olive oil to taste and toss.

Linguini and Mini-Burgers (A, O, P, S, L)

After putting filtered water on to boil, begin mini-burger preparation. Cook whole wheat, spinach or tomato linguini al dente.

Poultry Mini-Burgers (vegan recipe follows)

2 tablespoons olive oil

1 small onion finely chopped

1/2 cup stone ground whole wheat flour

1 tablespoon dried cilantro or oregano

1/4 teaspoon black pepper

1/4 teaspoon paprika

1/4 teaspoon sea salt

1/4 teaspoon turmeric

1 lb ground chicken or turkey

Lightly sauté onion in olive oil and remove from the flame. Preheat the oven to 325 degrees. Combine flour, cilantro, pepper, paprika, salt, and turmeric in a small bowl. Once the oil has cooled, mix it with the ground meat. Flatten the ground meat and sprinkle the flour and spice mixture on top. Knead it until evenly distributed. Shape into small spheres and flatten into mini-burgers. Place on baking sheet. Bake the mini-burgers for 20 minutes, or until light brown. Flip them over and bake another 15 to 20 minutes, or until well done.

Makes about 20 to 24 mini-burgers.

Add to tomato sauce and serve over linguini.

Mini-burgers can also be eaten as *Bright* snacks, on salad or in place of protein bars or whey for resistance training.

LEGEND
A = Antioxidant
O = Vital Oil
P = Smart Protein
S = Slowly-Absorbed Glucose
L = Lower in Additives or Toxins

Vegan Spheres

1/4 cup olive oil

1 small onion, finely chopped

2 cups kidney beans, cooked

1 cup wild rice, cooked

1 tablespoon mustard, ground

1 teaspoon black pepper

1 teaspoon sage, rubbed

1 teaspoon thyme, ground

1/4 teaspoon sea salt

1/4 cup pectin, liquid

2 tablespoons olive oil

Preheat oven to 350 degrees. Sauté the onions in oil until they start to brown, and remove from flame. Combine beans, rice, mustard, pepper, sage, thyme, salt, pectin, and oil. Using a potato masher, stir together and smash. Shape into small spheres about one inch in diameter (for firmer and more manageable results, add 1/4 to 1/2 cup stone ground whole wheat flour to bean mixture). Place on an oiled baking sheet, and spray each of the spheres with olive oil. Cook for 25 to 30 minutes, or until light brown.

Makes about 24 vegan spheres.

Serve over linguini, and top with tomato sauce.

Vegan spheres can also be eaten as *Bright* snacks, in wraps and subs, or on top of salad.

Chicken Tenders (A, O, P, S, L)

1 1/2 lbs chicken breasts

1/4 cup unbleached flour

1 teaspoon mustard, ground

1/2 teaspoon paprika

1/2 teaspoon turmeric

1/2 teaspoon white pepper

2 eggs

3 tablespoons filtered water or sherry

1 cup bread crumbs, all natural Japanese style or regular

olive oil mister

Preheat oven to 375 degrees. Carefully cut chicken breasts into short strips. Set up three bowls, the first containing flour mixed with mustard, paprika, turmeric, and pepper; the second containing beaten egg and water; and the third containing all natural regular or Japanese-style bread crumbs (see Internet Addresses). Coat the chicken tenders with flour, then egg, then bread crumbs. Place them on lightly oiled baking sheets. Bake for about 15 minutes and spray them with olive oil. Bake another ten to 15 minutes, or until they're almost light brown.

Makes 24 to 32.

Dips: catsup, guacamole, hummus or mustard

Chicken tenders can also be eaten as *Bright* snacks, or on salad or subs.

LEGEND
A = Antioxidant
O = Vital Oil
P = Smart Protein
S = Slowly-Absorbed Glucose
L = Lower in Additives or Toxins

Macaroni, Broccoli, and Cheese (A, O, P, S, L)

3 cups broccoli florets, coarsely chopped

8 ozs whole wheat macaroni

1/4 cup olive oil

4 tablespoons unbleached flour

1/4 teaspoon white pepper

2 1/2 cups fat free milk

1 1/2 cups shredded reduced fat sharp cheddar

When water for pasta boils, add the broccoli for one minute, then remove with a strainer spoon. Cook pasta al dente in the same water. Over a medium flame, heat a large sauce pan containing about an inch of water. Warm olive oil, flour, and pepper in a medium saucepan over another medium flame. Stir until flour is dissolved and cook, while stirring continuously for about two minutes. Slowly add milk and whisk continuously for four minutes. Place the medium saucepan containing milk inside the large sauce pan containing hot water as you would a double-boiler for about ten minutes, or until the mixture thickens, stirring frequently. Stir in the cheese until melted into a smooth sauce. Remove cheese sauce from the double boiler, and wipe the bottom with a towel. Mix cheese sauce with pasta and broccoli. Serves six to eight.

White Chili con Carne (A, O, P, S, L)

Soak navy beans as directed, or pour eight cups of filtered water in a drip coffee reservoir, and place the navy beans in the coffee pot. Place the coffee pot on its hot plate and turn on the coffee maker. Allow the beans to soak in hot water for an hour. Pour off the hot water, holding the beans back at the spout with a fork. Fill up the coffee pot with filtered water and rinse beans two more times. Cook beans in a large pot until tender and strain.

1/2 cup olive oil

1 onion finely chopped

1 tablespoon mustard ground

1 teaspoon chili powder

1/2 teaspoon white pepper

1/4 teaspoon sea salt

2 lbs ground chicken or turkey meat

3 cups navy beans, cooked

4 cups filtered water

In a large pot over a low flame, sauté onion, mustard, chili, pepper, and salt in olive oil. Add the ground meat and sauté on a medium flame until cooked, breaking up meat clumps frequently, and stirring. Add the cooked beans and water. Raise the flame and bring to a boil. Then simmer with the lid off for about 25 minutes. Serves six as an entrée in a soup bowl. It can also be served with a strainer spoon over wild rice, as a side dish or a *Bright* snack.

LEGEND
A = Antioxidant
O = Vital Oil
P = Smart Protein
S = Slowly-Absorbed Glucose
L = Lower in Additives or Toxins

Answers for white chili con carne:

Olive oil – A, O, L
Onion finely chopped – A, L
Mustard ground – A, L
Chili powder – A, L
White pepper – A, L
Sea salt – L
Ground chicken or turkey meat – P, L
Navy beans, cooked – A, O, P, S, L
Filtered water – L

Wild Rice, Corn, and Cashews (A, O, P, S, L)

1/2 cup olive oil

1 medium onion finely chopped

1/2 red pepper, diced

2 tablespoons parsley

2 tablespoons marjoram

1/2 teaspoon black pepper

1/2 teaspoon sea salt

1 cup wild rice

3 cups filtered water

1 cup corn

1/4 cup cashew halves, raw

In a medium pot over a medium flame, lightly sauté onion and red pepper in olive oil. Add parsley, marjoram, black pepper, salt, rice, and water, and cover. Bring to a boil and simmer for 30 minutes. Add corn and cashews and simmer uncovered for 15 minutes. Drain and serve.

Serves six to eight.

Steak (A, O, P, L)

"Brighter steak" means cooking lean cuts of beef medium-rare, leaving burnt protein on the side, and topping with a little olive oil. Ground meat must be cooked until it's well done.

Smashed Potatoes (A, O, P, S, L)

6 medium potatoes with cleaned skins

3 cups cauliflower, cubed

1/4 cup olive oil

1/2 cup fat free milk or filtered water

2 tablespoons hummus

1/4 teaspoon sea salt

Cut each potato into quarters keeping the skin on and boil for about 15 minutes, or until easily pierced by a fork. In a separate pot, boil cauliflower for about 15 minutes, or until well done. Drain each. Smash potatoes, and pour about 3/4 of the oil and about 3/4 of the milk over them; stir a few times. Add hummus and salt and the rest of the oil and milk to the cauliflower, and mash thoroughly. Stir the mashed cauliflower into the smashed potatoes.

Serves six.

Answers for smashed potatoes:

Medium potatoes with cleaned skins – A, L
Cauliflower, cubed – A, S, L
Olive oil – A, O, L
Fat free milk – P, S, L or filtered water – L
Hummus – A, O, P, S, L
Sea salt – L

LEGEND
A = Antioxidant
O = Vital Oil
P = Smart Protein
S = Slowly-Absorbed Glucose
L = Lower in Additives or Toxins

BAKERY

These recipes were designed for home use. Softer and puffier results are obtained by commercial bakers using molds and a "proofer," which is a temperature and humidity-controlled cabinet.

BrightFoods English Muffins (A, O, P, S, L)

1 1/4 cups warm filtered water

1 teaspoon maple syrup

1/4 teaspoon raw sugar

2 pkgs dry yeast

2 cups stone ground whole wheat flour

1/4 teaspoon sea salt

1 tablespoon olive oil

Combine water, syrup, sugar, and yeast in a container, and stir. Allow ten minutes for rising. Stir together the flour and salt in a medium bowl. Add yeast mixture to flour; using a tablespoon, stir together. Collect into a dough mass. Oil the bottom of the bowl. Flatten the dough and cut into eight slices, like a pizza. Place eight oiled English muffin rings onto a lightly oiled cookie sheet, and flour the inside of the rings. Collect each slice using a tablespoon, and place inside English muffin ring. Lightly flour the tops, and, using your fingertips, flatten each muffin to better fit the mold. Cover with a towel and allow rising for 15 minutes, or until double the size.

Preheat oven to 350 degrees. Bake for about 25 minutes, or until light brown. Allow to cool and use a knife around the inside of each mold to remove muffins.

Makes eight English muffins.

BrightFoods Burger Buns and Hot Dog Rolls (A, O, P, S, L)

3 pkgs dry yeast

1/4 teaspoon raw sugar

2 1/2 cups warm filtered water

1 teaspoon sea salt

3 tablespoons organic maple syrup

3 tablespoons olive oil

5 cups stone ground whole wheat flour

Stir yeast and sugar into water; let stand for ten minutes.

In a mixing bowl, combine two cups flour and salt. Stir a few times. Add the yeast to the flour and stir into a doughy paste. Add syrup and oil, and stir. Add three cups flour and mix by hand into dough. Remove the dough and knead on a well floured surface for about six minutes, or until smooth. Place in an oiled bowl then flip the dough over.

Burger Buns – Remove from bowl and cut into 12 pieces. Knead each piece until smooth, and shape into burger bun. Place the buns on oiled baking sheets (can use oiled English muffin rings as molds), and lay a towel on top. Allow to rise for 30 minutes, or until double.

Hot Dog Rolls – Remove from bowl and cut into four chunks. Roll each about 1 1/2 inches thick and 15 inches long. Cut each of the four cylinders into three pieces. Shape each piece into a hot dog roll. Place the rolls on an oiled baking sheet (best results with commercial mold and proofer); lay towel on top. Allow to rise for 30 minutes, or until doubled in size.

Preheat oven to 350 degrees and bake the rolls for about 35 to 40 minutes, or until light brown; spray the tops with water every ten minutes.

Makes 12 rolls or buns.

LEGEND
A = Antioxidant
O = Vital Oil
P = Smart Protein
S = Slowly-Absorbed Glucose
L = Lower in Additives or Toxins

BrightFoods Grain Buns with Orange and Cinnamon (A, O, P, S, L)

2 pkgs active dry yeast

1/4 teaspoon raw sugar

1 cup warm filtered water

2 cups orange juice

1/2 cup orange marmalade

1/4 cup olive oil

1 egg

1 cup old fashioned oats

1/2 cup raw sugar

1 teaspoon cinnamon

1/2 teaspoon sea salt

6 cups stone ground whole wheat flour

Dissolve yeast and sugar in water and allow to stand for about five minutes. In a small sauce pan, combine juice, marmalade, oil, and egg, and beat together. Warm the mixture on a medium flame for three minutes, then remove from the flame. In a medium bowl, combine oats, one of the cups of flour, sugar, cinnamon, and salt. Add yeast mixture to flour, and stir for about one minute. Add orange mixture and stir for about two minutes. Whisk for about a minute. Stir in remaining five cups of flour. Flatten dough in a floured bowl. Flour the top and cover with plastic wrap and a towel; allow to rise for 30 minutes, or until double the size.

1/2 cup raw sugar

2 tablespoons cinnamon

6 tablespoons olive oil

Mister

Mix sugar and cinnamon. Flatten dough on a well-floured surface and cut into two equal pieces. Dust with flour and roll into rectangles, each about 15 x 9 inches. Brush with olive oil and sprinkle with the sugar/cinnamon mix. Roll up the long side of each, seal edge closed with water, and pinch. Flour the surface again and roll and shape the cylinders symmetrically.

Cut each roll into 12 slices and place slices spiral face up in oiled muffin pans. Press bun to fill up the bottom half of each muffin mold. Spray the tops with olive oil. Cover and let rise for 40 minutes, or until doubled in size. Preheat oven to 375 degrees and bake for 20 to 25 minutes, spraying them with water every ten minutes, or until buns are light brown. Eat plain, or top with orange marmalade or Nutella.

Makes 24 buns.

About the Chef

These recipes and the ones in *The BrightFoods Cookbook* were developed and tested by Dr. Cocores. Does he have any "chef" experience? Dr. Cocores' familiarity with kitchens and cooking started at the age of five. As a student in elementary school and the first member of a dual-income family to arrive home on weekday afternoons, he usually started dinner by putting a pot of water on for spaghetti. In his household, it wasn't uncommon to host multi-entrée dinner parties like the ones portrayed in *My Big Fat Greek Wedding*, or to reciprocate to gatherings of similar magnitude.

A close family friend was a medical school nutrition professor, and this physician had a major influence on Dr. Cocores' early awareness of the links between food and the body. At the same time, cooking rapidly became a hobby, and by the age of 13 he'd landed his first job outside the home washing bakery pots and sheets. Within a year, he became a baker's assistant. Years later he secured working papers and started stocking shelves, unloading trucks and bagging items in one of the supermarkets owned by a family friend. He went on to manage and order items for four grocery aisles.

Because a mild reading disability made it hard for him to follow recipes, he has been creating his own recipes since the age of 16. To this day, when dining out, he tries to figure out the ingredients in different dishes and baked goods. (For more information about the origins of *BrightFoods*, see Appendix V.)

Now that you have some idea of the scope of our sample menus and corresponding recipes, and a little background about the chef himself, let's take a look at some of the *BrightFoods* programs.

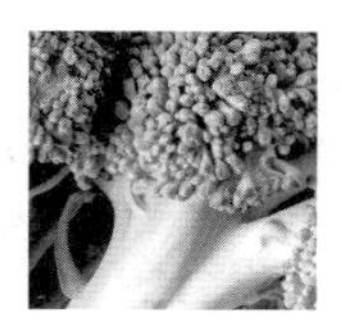

CHAPTER TEN
BrightFoods Programs – From Text to Table

Revolutions begin one person at a time.

We believe that this book offers the most comprehensive analysis available of how foods potentially impact brain cells, learning, memory, mood, and performance. The *BrightFoods* eating plan can help brain cells and the mind function more efficiently. It also tells you how to provide vital nutrients to other organs, help your waistline, and extend your life. *BrightFoods* creates innovative nutritional programs designed to help improve mental focus, behavior, weight control, and overall health. Because it goes well beyond most plans for "healthy" eating and requires commitment to follow, it may take some time before the *BrightFoods* lifestyle becomes mainstream. In the meantime, here's how you can get started.

At Home

Start with some of the recipes in the *BrightFoods* Sample Menus. If you'd like more, you'll want to get the *BrightFoods Cookbook*, a collection of all-American favorites and dishes from 12 different countries. Since some of the recipes for home-made baked goods require kneading, you may want to get a bread-maker; if no one volunteers (just kidding), consider buying an affordable model. Or if you'd prefer not to, you can pick up slowly-absorbed breads from the grocery store.

If ordering home delivery is your idea of cooking, contact Psyche Nutrition Sciences, Inc., for availability in your area.

Schools

"Low fat," "low carb," and "diet" are just some of the catchy phrases that have helped to aggravate a nutrition problem in America. But with *BrightFoods*, it's possible for our students to eat their way to better health and improved performance.

Private schools – The first step includes nutritional education for administrators, students, staff, and parents, followed by evaluation and the development of nutritional standards and policies. We also provide guidance to help create a self-administering nutrition committee within each school, develop menus, and select qualified food vendors. We arrange for meal delivery management, with ongoing regulatory compliance oversight and quality assurance, and provide supporting products and informational materials, as well as counseling and assistance on fundraising and financial issues.

Private universities and colleges – We bring information about brightening up campus cafeterias to the dean of students, and offer the same support to institutions of higher learning as we do to private schools.

Public schools, county colleges, and state universities are more dependent on county, state, and federal funds to balance their budgets. Here, brightening up the school cafeteria may require increasing the cost of the lunch meal and/or working with local legislators. Psyche Nutrition Sciences can provide guidance about the *BrightFoods* eating concept to board of education members, governors, congressmen, and senators.

Healthcare Facilities

It's a well-known yet often overlooked fact that proper nutrition is vital to anyone with health issues. This is especially true when it comes to the elderly. They're the ones who're most at risk for developing medical problems, chronic illnesses, the flu, colds, pneumonia, and general failing health. It's unfortunate that commercial interests have promoted fad diets to the extent that most people are grossly misinformed about the science of nutrition. But it is possible for those with health issues, including the elderly, to eat their way to better health and improved mental performance.

The *BrightFoods* plan can find its way into assisted living, halfway houses, hospitals, nursing homes, partial hospitalization programs, and substance abuse treatment facilities. For example, Psyche Nutrition Sciences is currently serving as consultant to Patient Care Management Associates, a concierge medicine service provider that helps doctors offer more efficient treatment to their clients.

Business

Businesses are suffering from ever-increasing healthcare costs, as they cover expenses incurred by employee obesity, hypertension, absenteeism, and lack of energy. The problem isn't so much that workers don't have access to proper healthcare as it is that there's general apathy towards a proactive approach to good health. The *BrightFoods* program includes nutritional education for mid-level executives and their employees, and the establishment of internal nutritional standards and policies tailored to the workplace. We also provide guidance to create a self-administering advisory committee, menus, and vendor selections. In addition, we offer a qualification program to ensure that appropriate meals and snacks are delivered, and make sure that staffs have supporting products and information.

Food Manufacturers

BrightFoods offers consultation services to manufacturers of:

- Baked goods
- Baking products
- Bread, buns, rolls, wraps
- Frozen foods and pizza
- Grocery items
- Pasta
- Peanut butter
- Supplements

Restaurants

Consultative services are also available to:

- Franchise bakeries
- Franchise juiceries
- Franchise pizzerias
- Franchise restaurants
- Franchise retailers with food bars
- Hotels

Research and Development

The *BrightFoods* research and development program keeps abreast of the latest information and findings at the mind/nutrition interface. We stay current, as we demonstrate in our medical source citations; about half of the close to 900 contained in this book are less than two years old. In addition, we compare the data collected from schools, workplaces, and healthcare settings to outcome and follow-up studies.

For more information about Psyche Nutrition Sciences, visit us at **www.PNSI-Inc.com**.

APPENDIX I

BrightFoods Pyramid

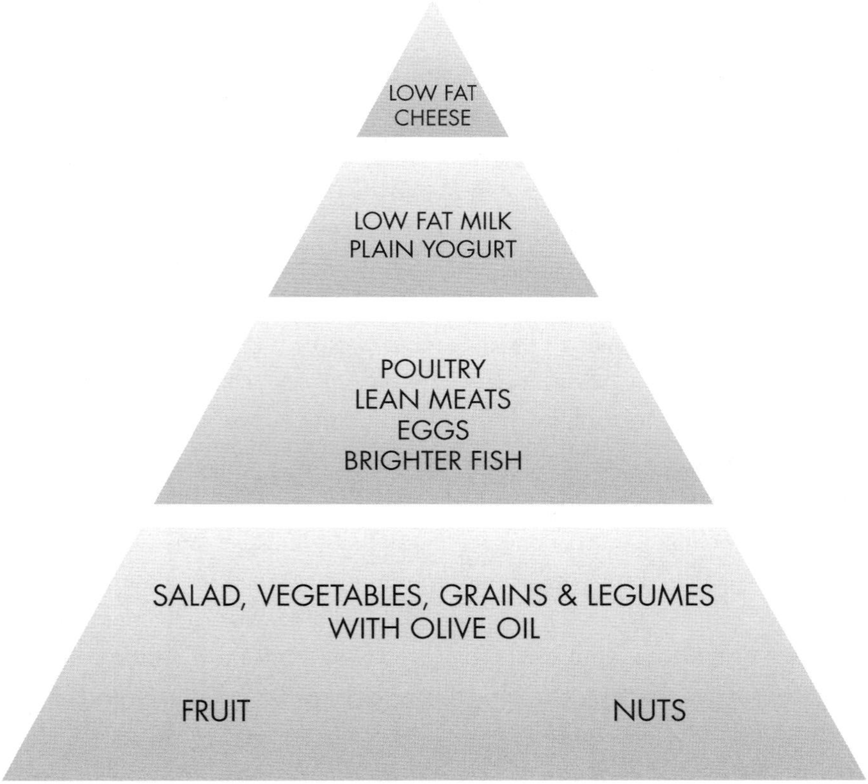

LOW FAT
CHEESE

LOW FAT MILK
PLAIN YOGURT

POULTRY
LEAN MEATS
EGGS
BRIGHTER FISH

SALAD, VEGETABLES, GRAINS & LEGUMES
WITH OLIVE OIL

FRUIT NUTS

APPENDIX II
Fish School

These conservative guidelines were established by Dr. Cocores, an avid deep sea and freshwater fisherman, in response to numerous patient questions and requests. The charts that follow were based on information compiled from a number of scientific sources, including the US Department of Health and Human Services and the US Environmental Protection Agency (http://www.cfsan.fda.gov/~frf/sea-mehg.html). Dr. Cocores also drew on the mercury (Hg) and dioxin medical journal sources listed for Chapter Five, as well as his own laboratory testing of tuna and swordfish to formulate the ratings and guidelines below. It hasn't been proven that using these guidelines leads to better health than not using them. This chart in no way reflects the opinions or advice set forth by the US Department of Health and Human Services and the US Environmental Protection Agency. They're merely the author's opinion as to how the health-conscious can manage their fish consumption. He intends no implicit criticism of the fish industry; rather, he hopes to give his readers the facts, and allow them to decide for themselves.

G-Rated Fish contain 0.00 ppm (parts per million) mercury. We set no limits on clam, ocean perch, shrimp, or whiting consumption, providing it's served as part of a balanced meal or snack to people without cholesterol problems, sensitivity to sulfite or benzoate, and with their physician's approval. Canned salmon is approved for people over 18 twice weekly when eaten along with antioxidant and 500 mgs vitamin C, and in children ten to 18 once per week when accompanied by antioxidant and 250 mgs of Ester C, with pediatrician approval.

Species	High in Cholesterol	Potentially High in Dioxin
Clam	YES	Not a Problem
Ocean Perch	Not a Problem	Not a Problem
Salmon, canned (D)	Not a Problem	YES
Shrimp (S)	YES	Not a Problem
Whiting	Not a Problem	Not a Problem

D – Potentially contains higher levels of PBCs and other dioxins when compared to other fish due to higher fat content.

S – Conventional fish, especially shrimp, may contain sulfites and benzoates, which may not be present in organic fish.

PG-10 Fish – Adults older than 18 may choose two servings per week, taken along with bioavailable antioxidants and 500 mgs vitamin C. Children between the ages of ten and 18 may eat one serving every two weeks when taken along with bioavailable antioxidants and 250 mgs of Ester C, if pediatrician approved.

Species	Mercury in PPM	Potentially High in Dioxin
Anchovies	0.04	YES
Herring	0.04	YES
Flounder or Sole	0.04	
Haddock	0.03	
Crawfish (C)	0.03	
Sardine	0.02	YES
Oyster (C)	0.01	
Talapia	0.01	
Hake	0.01	
Salmon, fresh	0.01	YES

C – Possibly high in cholesterol.

PG-18 Fish – Adults older than 18 may choose one serving per week, taken along with bioavailable antioxidants or 500 mgs vitamin C. Children between the ages of ten and 18 may eat one serving per month, taken along with bioavailable antioxidants and 250 mgs Ester C, with a pediatrician's approval. Not recommended for pregnant or lactating mothers.

Species	Hg in PPM	Species	Hg in PPM
Lobster, spiny (C)	0.09	Butterfish	0.06
Mackerel, chub (D)	0.09	Crab (C)	0.06
Whitefish (D)	0.07	Catfish	0.05
Croaker, Atlantic	0.07	Mullet (D)	0.05
Trout, freshwater Trout, lake (D)	0.07	Flatfish	0.05
Shad	0.07	Mackerel, Atlantic (D)	0.05
Squid (C)	0.07	Scallop (C)	0.05

C – Possibly high in cholesterol.

D – Potentially contains higher levels of PBCs and other dioxins when compared to other fish.

R Rated Fish – Adults older than 18 may choose one serving every two weeks, when served with plenty of bioavailable antioxidants and 1000 mg vitamin C. Not recommended in pregnant or lactating mothers, or children under the age of 18.

Species	Hg	Species	Hg
Bass, Chilean	0.39	Snapper	0.19
Tuna, fresh albacore	0.36	Mahi Mahi	0.19
Tuna, canned	0.35	Monkfish	0.18
Bluefish (D)	0.34	Mackerel, Spanish	0.18
Tuna, fresh yellowfin	0.33	Tilefish, Atlantic	0.14
Lobster, N. Amer. (C)	0.31	Perch, freshwater	0.14
Croaker, white	0.29	Carp	0.14
Scorpionfish	0.29	Skate	0.14
Weakfish – Sea Trout	0.26	Sheepshead	0.13
Halibut	0.25	Tuna, canned	0.12
Bass, saltwater	0.22	Jacksmelt	0.11
Sablefish (D)	0.22	Cod	0.10
Tuna, fresh Skipjack	0.21		

D – Potentially contains higher levels of PBC's and other dioxins when compared with other fish.
C – Possibly high in cholesterol.

Not Rated or Recommended

Species	Hg in PPM	Species	Hg in PPM
Tilefish, Gulf of Mexico	1.45	Orange Roughy	0.55
Shark	0.99	Marlin	0.49
Swordfish	0.98	Grouper	0.47
Mackerel, king (D)	0.73	Mackerel, Spanish, Gulf of Mexico (D)	0.45
Tuna, fresh bigeye	0.64		

D – Potentially contains higher levels of PBC's and other dioxins when compared to other fish.

APPENDIX III:
Glucose Absorption Rate for Various Foods

Slowly Absorbed (SA) Glucose – The Best Carbs

FRUIT

Apple
Banana
Cherry
Fig
Grapefruit
Grape, green
Mango
Orange
Peach
Pear
Plum
Prune
Strawberry, organic

JUICE, unsweetened

Apple
Carrot
Grapefruit
Pineapple
Tomato

SOUP, low additive

Lentil
Minestrone
Tomato

NUTS, unsalted

Almond
Brazil Nut
Cashew
Peanut (legume)
Pecan
Macadamia
Walnut

VEGETABLES

Artichoke
Asparagus
Avocado
Broccoli
Cabbage
Carrot
Cauliflower
Celery
Corn
Cucumber
Eggplant
Garlic
Green Bean
Lettuce
Mushroom
Pea
Pepper
Potato Dumpling
Smashed Potato ala *Bright*
Spinach
Squash
Sweet Potato
Zucchini

LEGUMES

Black Bean
Blackeyed Pea
Butter Bean
Cannellini
Chickpeas
Hummus
Kidney Bean
Lentils
Mung Bean Noodles
Navy
Pinto
Split Peas

GRAIN

Bulgar
Barley, not instant
Converted Rice
Fettuccine
Koshikari Rice
Linguni
Macaroni
Pastina
Rice Bran
Spaghetti
Spirali
Vermicelli
Wild Rice

BREAD

Buckwheat
Cracked Wheat
9 Grain or Greater
Oat Bran
Pumpernickle
Sourdough
Sourdough Rye
Stoneground Wheat 100%

CEREAL

Kelloggs Complete Oat
Kelloggs Complete Wheat
Old Fashioned Oatmeal
Zone Breakfast Cereal

All tables extrapolated from works by Jennie Brand-Miller, Johanna Burani, and Kaye Foster-Powell, Australia.

Non Essential Sources of Slowly Absorbed (SA) Glucose

SPREADS

Nutella
Orange Marmalade
Peanut Butter
Strawberry Jam, organic

DAIRY

Chocolate Ice Cream
Low Fat Chocolate Milk
Vanilla Ice Milk
Skim Milk
Yogurt, plain

FROZEN

Ravioli, meat
Tortellini, cheese

SWEETNERS

Fructose
Lactose
Maple Syrup
Real Maple Syrup, Organic

PUDDING

Chocolate
Vanilla

MOUSSE

Berry
Butterscotch
Chocolate
Hazelnut
Mango
Strawberry, organic

COOKIES

Crème Filled Wafers
Social Tea Biscuits
Twix Bar, carmel

CAKE or MUFFIN

Apple
Banana
Chocolate
Pound
Sponge
Strawberry Short
Vanilla

CANDY

Dark Chocolate
M&M Peanut

Moderately Absorbed (MA) Glucose Sources – Not For Overweight or Diabetic People

Angel Food Cake
Angel Hair Pasta (ef)
Apricot
Banana Muffin (ef)
Basmati Rice (B)
Beet
Black Bean Soup
Blueberry Muffin (ef)
Bran Buds Cereal (B)
Bran Chex (B)
Bran Muffin (ef)
Brown Rice
Cantaloupe
Coca-Cola (B)
Condensed Milk
Corn Meal
Couscous
Cranberry Juice
Cream of Wheat (B)
Croissant (ef)
French Baguette (ef) + spreads
Frosted Flakes (B)
Gnocchi (ef)
Granola Bar
Grapenuts Cereal (B)
Green Pea Soup
Hamburger Bun (ef)
Kudos Granola Bar (B)
Life Cereal (B)
Long Grain Rice
Low Fat Vanilla Ice Cream
Macaroni & Cheese, box
Mars Bar (B)
Mini Wheats (B)
Oat Bran Muffin (ef)
Orange Juice, carton (B)
Papaya
Peach, canned
Pineapple
Potato, no oil or vinegar
Power Bar (B)
Quick Oats (B)
Raisins
Rice Noodles
Rice Vermicelli
Snickers (B)
Risotto
Rye Bread
Shredded Wheat (B)
Smacks Cereal (B)
Special K (B)
Split Pea Soup
Stoned Wheat Thins (B)
Table Sugar (sucrose)
Taco Shell
Thin Linguine (ef)
Whole Grain Bread

ef – Made with white enriched flour.

B – Extrapolated from works by Jennie Brand-Miller, Johanna Burani, and Kaye Foster-Powell, Australia.

Rapidly Absorbed (RA) Glucose Sources – Not Recommended

Bagel, plain or whole wheat (ef)
Bran Flakes (B)
Cheerios (B)
Corn Chips
Corn Flakes (B)
Corn Muffin
Corn Pops (B)
Cupcake (ef)
Date, dried
Doughnut
English Muffin (ef) no butter
Fava Bean
French Baguette (ef) no butter
French Fries
Fruit Roll-ups (B)
Gatorade (B)
Glucose Tablets
Golden Grahams Cereal (B)
Fructose Corn Syrup
Instant Mashed Potato
Instant Rice
Jasmine Rice
Jelly Beans
Life Savers (B)
Pop Corn
Pop Tarts (B)
Pretzels (ef)
Puffed Wheat Cereal (B)
Pumpkin, mashed
Raisin Bran (B)
Rice Cakes
Rice Chex (B)
Rice Crispies (B)
Rutabaga
Saltine Crackers (B)
Scones (ef)
Skittles (B)
Tapioca Pudding
Tofu Frozen Dessert (B)
Total Cereal (B)
Vanilla Wafers (B)
Watermelon
White Bread (ef)
Whole Wheat Bread (ef)

ef – Made with white enriched flourB – extrapolated from works by Jennie Brand-Miller, Johanna Burani, and Kaye Foster-Powell, Australia.

B – Extrapolated from works by Jennie Brand-Miller, Johanna Burani, and Kaye Foster-Powell, Australia.

APPENDIX IV

Not Uncommon Drinking and Bottled Water Contaminants Found in Tiny Amounts

- Microorganisms such as fecal coliform, *E. coli*, Cryptosporidium, and *Giardia lamblia*
- Radioactive minerals including alpha emitters, beta/photon emitters, radium, and radon
- Inorganic matter including asbestos, arsenic, cyanide, fluoride, lead, mercury, and thallium
- Organic matter such as pesticides and herbicides, including, but not limited to: acrylamide, atrazine, dioxin, ethylene dibromide, PCBs or polychlorinated biphenyls, pentachlorophenol, and toxaphene
- Germicides and byproducts such as chlorine, chloramines, chlorine dioxide, trihalomethanes, haloacetic acids, bromate, and chlorite
- A gasoline additive used to make auto emissions cleaner called MTBE

APPENDIX V
The Roots of *BrightFoods* Eating: An Overview of Nutritional Neuropsychiatry

This appendix explains, to readers who are curious, how *BrightFoods* was developed for addicts in recovery, and shows why it benefits the general population as well.

BrightFoods finds its roots in the "The Sobriety Diet," conceived by Dr. Cocores in 1985 and published in 1990 as part of his *800-COCAINE Book of Drug and Alcohol Recovery*. A version of "The Sobriety Diet" tailored for smokers appeared in his 1991 textbook, *The Clinical Management of Nicotine Dependence*. The diet was fashioned to help reduce alcohol and drug cravings, and has been presented to more than 30,000 patients since 1985. It's been continually updated, and used in conjunction with therapy and medicine to treat every psychiatric condition known.

Dr. Cocores has used *The Mood Diet* handout, an outline of *BrightFoods: Discover the surprising link between food and learning, memory, mood, and performance*, from 2001 until 2005 to treat thousands of patients. In 2003 he redirected his research activities from spiritual psychiatry which began on 9/11 to writing a *Mood Diet* pamphlet to support lessons touched on during psychotherapy. That pamphlet forms the basis of this book.

Medicinal foods are important additions to treatment. *BrightFoods* wasn't designed to replace psychotherapy and psychopharmacology. In general, *BrightFoods* can make therapy more productive, accelerate the process and help medicines for the mind work better. But it doesn't replace any of these treatments, taken together or separately.

In conjunction with psychotherapy and medication, *BrightFoods* has been found to calm many of the symptoms psychiatric patients experience, and to ease or eliminate many of the less-intense psychiatric and psychosomatic symptoms and behaviors experienced by the general population, including:

- addictions, aggression, anxiety, apathy, autism, attention deficit
- cravings for carbohydrates, cheese, chips, chocolate, cookies, cakes and ice cream, compulsions, concentration problems, cramping, crying

- day-dreaming, dizziness, depression, evening bingeing
- fatigue, fears, fibromyalgia, forgetfulness
- grinding teeth, headaches, hunger, hyperactivity, hypersomnia, hypertension, hopelessness, indifference, impulsivity, insomnia, irritability, irritable bowl syndrome, lack of energy, laziness, decreased sex drive, learning disabilities
- memory problems, mental confusion or exhaustion, mood changes and swings
- nail biting, nervousness, muscle tightness, obsessions, over-sensitivity, panic feelings, paranoia, phobias, PMS, restlessness, rituals
- seasonal blues, shallow sleeping, shortness of breath, shyness, spacey feelings, suicidal thoughts
- tension, tiredness that's prolonged, unreal feelings, and worrying

Addictive foods can cause or intensify all these symptoms, and more.

MEDICAL JOURNAL SOURCES

CHAPTER ONE: How Healthy Brain Cells Help Us Learn

Bianchi M, Hagan JJ, Heidbreder CA, Brain cellal plasticity, stress and depression: involvement of the cytoskeletal microtubular system? *Curr Drug Targets CNS Neurol Disord.* Oct;4(5):597-611, 2005

Brunson KL, Chen Y, Avishai-Eliner S, Stress and the developing hippocampus: a double-edged sword? *Mol Neurobiol.* Apr;27(2):121-36, 2003

Burke SN, Barnes CA, Neural plasticity in the ageing brain. *Nat Rev Neurosci.* Jan;7(1):30-40, 2006

Cotman CW, Berchtold NC, Exercise: a behavioral intervention to enhance brain health and plasticity. *Trends Neurosci.* Jun;25(6):295-301, 2002

Guo Q, When good Cdk5 turns bad. *Sci Aging Knowledge Environ.* Feb8;(5), 2006

Jay TM, Rocher C, Hotte M, et al, Plasticity at hippocampal to prefrontal cortex synapses is impaired by loss of dopamine and stress: importance for psychiatric diseases. *Neurotox Res.* 6(3):233-44, 2004

Kim JJ, Diamond DM, The stressed hippocampus, synaptic plasticity and lost memories. *Nat Rev Neurosci.* Jun;3(6):453-62, 2002

Kleim JA, Jones TA, Schallert T, Motor enrichment and the induction of plasticity before or after brain injury. *Neurochem Res.* Nov;28(11):1757-69, 2003

Kolb B, Whishaw IQ, Brain plasticity and behavior. *Annu Rev Psychol.* 49:43-64, 1998

Lazar SW, Kerr CE, Wasserman RH, et al, Meditation experience is associated with increased cortical thickness. *Neuroreport.* Nov 28;16(17):1893-7, 2005

Lou HC, Nowak M, Kjaer TW, The mental self. *Prog Brain Res.* 150:197-204, 2005

Maguire EA, Spiers HJ, Good CD, et al, Navigation expertise and the human hippocampus: a structural brain imaging analysis. *Hippocampus.* 13(2):250-9, 2003

McEwen BS, Glucocorticoids, depression, and mood disorders: structural remodeling in the brain. *Metabolism.* May;54(5 Suppl 1):20-3, 2005

Milad MR, Quinn BT, Pitman RK, et al, Thickness of ventromedial prefrontal cortex in humans is correlated with extinction memory. *Proc Natl Acad Sci USA.* Jul 26;102(30):10706-11, 2005

Newberg A, Alavi A, Baime M, et al, The measurement of regional cerebral blood flow during the complex cognitive task of meditation: a preliminary SPECT study. *Psychiatry Res.* Apr 10;106(2):113-22, 2001

Radley JJ, Morrison JH, Repeated stress and structural plasticity in the brain. *Ageing Res Rev.* May;4(2):271-87, 2005

Sapolsky RM, Stress and plasticity in the limbic system. *Neurochem Res.* Nov;28(11):1735-42, 2003

Siegel DJ, An Interpersonal Neurobiology Approach to Psychotherapy. *Psychiatric Annals.* 36;4, 248-56, 2006

Travis F, Tecce JJ, Guttman J, Cortical plasticity, contingent negative variation, and transcendent experiences during practice of the Transcendental Meditation technique. *Biol Psychol.* Nov;55(1):41-55, 2000

Viamontes GI, Beitman BD, Neural Substrates of Psychotherapeutic Change: Part I. *Psychiatric Annals.* 36;4, 225-36, 2006

Viamontes GI, Beitman BD, Neural Substrates of Psychotherapeutic Change: Part II. *Psychiatric Annals.* 36;4, 238-46, 2006

Walker MP, Stickgold R, Sleep, memory, and plasticity. *Annu Rev Psychol.* 57:139-66, 2006

Xu J, Kang J, The mechanisms and functions of activity-dependent long-term potentiation of intrinsic excitability. *Rev Neurosci.* 16(4):311-23, 2005

CHAPTER TWO: Brain Cells Work for *BrightFoods*: How Food Affects Learning, Memory, Mood, and Performance

Baydas G, Ozveren F, Akdemir I, et al, Learning and memory deficits in rats induced by chronic thinner exposure are reversed by melatonin. *J Pineal Res.* Aug;39(1):50-6, 2005

Bazan NG, Lipid signaling in neural plasticity, brain repair, and neuroprotection. *Mol Neurobiol.* Aug;32(1):89-103, 2005

Benes FM, Taylor JB, Cunningham MC, Convergence and plasticity of monoaminergic systems in the medial prefrontal cortex during the postnatal period: implications for the development of psychopathology. *Cereb Cortex.* Oct;10(10):1014-27, 2000

Cole-Edwards KK, Bazan NG, Lipid signaling in experimental epilepsy. *Neurochem Res.* Jun-Jul; 30(6-7):847-53, 2005

Darlington CL, Astrocytes as targets for neuroprotective drugs. *Curr Opin Investig Drugs.* Jul; 6(7):700-3, 2005

de Jesus Ferreira MC, Crouzin N, Barbanel G, A transient treatment of hippocampal brain cells with alpha-tocopherol induces a long-lasting protection against oxidative damage via a genomic action. *Free Radic Biol Med.* Oct 15;39(8):1009-20, 2005

Douglas SJ, Dawson-Scully K, Sokolowski MB, The neurogenetics and evolution of food-related behaviour. *Trends Neurosci.* Dec;28(12):644-52, 2005

Hayley S, Poulter MO, Merali Z, et al, The pathogenesis of clinical depression: stressor- and cytokine-induced alterations of neuroplasticity. *Neuroscience.* 135(3):659-78, 2005

Hillard CJ, Lipids and drugs of abuse. *Life Sci.* Aug 19;77(14):1531-42, 2005

Horrocks LA, Farooqui AA, Docosahexaenoic acid in the diet: its importance in maintenance and restoration of neural membrane function. *Prostaglandins Leukot Essent Fatty Acids.* Apr;70(4):361-72, 2004

Horvath TL, The hardship of obesity: a soft-wired hypothalamus. *Nat Neurosci.* May;8(5):561-5, 2005

Kelley AE, Baldo BA, Pratt WE, et al, Corticostriatal-hypothalamic circuitry and food motivation: integration of energy, action and reward. *Physiol Behav.* Dec 15;86(5):773-95, 2005

Lau FC, Shukitt-Hale B, Joseph JA, The beneficial effects of fruit polyphenols on brain aging. *Neurobiol Aging.* Dec;26 Suppl 1:128-32, 2005

Mattson MP, Energy intake, meal frequency, and health: a neurobiological perspective. *Annu Rev Nutr.* 25:237-60, 2005

Mattson MP, Gene-diet interactions in brain aging and neurodegenerative disorders. *Ann Intern Med.* Sep 2;139(5 Pt 2):441-4, 2003

Mattson MP, Chan SL, Duan W, Modification of brain aging and neurodegenerative disorders by genes, diet, and behavior. *Physiol Rev.* Jul;82(3):637-72, 2002

Mattson MP, Duan W, Guo Z, Meal size and frequency affect brain cellal plasticity and vulnerability to disease: cellular and molecular mechanisms. *J Neurochem.* Feb;84(3):417-31, 2003

Molteni R, Wu A, Vaynman S, et al, Exercise reverses the harmful effects of consumption of a high-fat diet on synaptic and behavioral plasticity associated to the action of brain-derived neurotrophic factor. *Neuroscience.* 123(2):429-40, 2004

Nakamichi N, Oikawa H, Kambe Y, et al, Relevant modulation by ferrous ions of N-methyl-D-aspartate receptors in ischemic brain injuries. *Curr Neurovasc Res.* Dec;1(5):429-40, 2004

Salamone JD, Correa M, Mingote SM, et al, Beyond the reward hypothesis: alternative functions of nucleus accumbens dopamine. *Curr Opin Pharmacol.* Feb;5(1):34-41, 2005

Tapiero H, Mathe G, Couvreur P, et al, II. Glutamine and glutamate. *Biomed Pharmacother.* Nov;56(9):446-57, 2002

Thetford Smothers C, Woodward JJ, Effects of amino acid substitutions in transmembrane domains of the NR1 subunit on the ethanol inhibition of recombinant N-methyl-D-aspartate receptors. *Alcohol Clin Exp Res.* Mar;30(3):523-30, 2006

Wu A, Ying Z, Gomez-Pinilla F, Dietary curcumin counteracts the outcome of traumatic brain injury on oxidative stress, synaptic plasticity, and cognition. *Exp Neurol.* Feb;197(2):309-17, 2006

CHAPTER THREE: Brighten Your Mind: Reduce Brain Rust

Free Radicals, Oxidative Stress and the Brain

Albers DS, Beal MF, Mitochondrial dysfunction and oxidative stress in aging and neurodegenerative disease. *J Neural Transm Suppl.* 59:133-54, 2000

Beal MF, Oxidative damage as an early marker of Alzheimer's disease and mild cognitive impairment. *Neurobiol Aging.* May;26(5):585-6,2005

Beckman KB, Ames BN, Oxidative decay of DNA. *J Biol Chem.* Aug 8;272(32):19633-6, 1997

Butterfield DA, Howard BJ, LaFontaine MA., Brain oxidative stress in animal models of accelerated aging and the age-related neurodegenerative disorders, Alzheimer's disease and Huntington's disease. *Curr Med Chem.* Jun;8(7):815-28, 2001

Butterfield DA, Poon HF, St Clair D, et al, Redox proteomics identification of oxidatively modified hippocampal proteins in mild cognitive impairment: Insights into the development of Alzheimer's disease. *Neurobiol Dis.* Feb 6, 2006

Calabrese V, Lodi R, Tonon C, et al, Oxidative stress, mitochondrial dysfunction and cellular stress response in Friedreich's ataxia. *J Neurol Sci.* Jun 15;233(1-2):145-62, 2005

Calabrese V, Scapagnini G, Colombrita C, et al, Redox regulation of heat shock protein expression in aging and neurodegenerative disorders associated with oxidative stress: a nutritional approach. *Amino Acids.* Dec;25(3-4):437-44, 2003

Facheris M, Beretta S, Ferrarese C, Peripheral markers of oxidative stress and excitotoxicity in neurodegenerative disorders: tools for diagnosis and therapy? *J Alzheimers Dis.* Apr;6(2):177-84, 2004

Fukui K, Takatsu H, Shinkai T, et al. Appearance of amyloid beta-like substances and delayed-type apoptosis in rat hippocampus CA1 region through aging and oxidative stress. *J Alzheimers Dis.* Dec;8(3):299-309, 2005

Keller JN, Schmitt FA, Scheff SW, et al, Evidence of increased oxidative damage in subjects with mild cognitive impairment. *Neurology.* Apr 12;64(7):1152-6, 2005

Mariani E, Polidori MC, Cherubini A, et al. Oxidative stress in brain aging, neurodegenerative and vascular diseases: an overview. J Chromatogr B Analyt Technol Biomed *Life Sci.* Nov 15;827(1):65-75, 2005

Mattson MP, Metal-catalyzed disruption of membrane protein and lipid signaling in the pathogenesis of neurodegenerative disorders. *Ann N Y Acad Sci.* Mar;1012:37-50, 2004

Mattson MP, Haughey NJ, Nath A, Cell death in HIV dementia. *Cell Death Differ.* Aug;12 Suppl 1:893-904, 2005

Rabin BM, Shukitt-Hale B, Joseph J, et al. Diet as a factor in behavioral radiation protection following exposure to heavy particles. *Gravit Space Biol Bull.* Jun;18(2):71-7, 2005

Reddy PH, Amyloid precursor protein-mediated free radicals and oxidative damage: implications for the development and progression of Alzheimer's disease. *J Neurochem.* Jan;96(1):1-13, 2006

Sachdev PS, Anstey KJ, Parslow RA, et al, Pulmonary Function, Cognitive Impairment and Brain Atrophy in a Middle-Aged Community Sample. *Dement Geriatr Cogn Disord.* Feb 10;21(5-6):300-308, 2006

Schipper HM, Bennett DA, Liberman A, et al, Glial heme oxygenase-1 expression in Alzheimer disease and mild cognitive impairment. *Neurobiol Aging.* Feb;27(2):252-61, 2006

Solfrizzi V, D'Introno A, Colacicco AM, et al, Circulating biomarkers of cognitive decline and dementia. *Clin Chim Acta.* Feb;364(1-2):91-112, 2006

Free Radicals and Cardiovascular Disease

Chisolm GM, Steinberg D, The oxidative modification hypothesis of atherogenesis: an overview. *Free Radic Biol Med.* Jun 15;28(12):1815-26, 2000

Colles SM, Maxson JM, Carlson SG et al, Oxidized LDL-induced injury and apoptosis in atherosclerosis. Potential roles for oxysterols. *Trends Cardiovasc Med.* Apr-May;11(3-4):131-8,2001

Pollock DM, Pollock JS, Endothelin and oxidative stress in the vascular system. *Curr Vasc Pharmacol.* Oct;3(4):365-7, 2005

Free Radicals, Diabetes and Its Complications

Maritim AC, Sanders RA, Watkins JB 3rd. Diabetes, oxidative stress, and antioxidants: a review. *J Biochem Mol Toxicol.* 17(1):24-38, 2003

Osawa T, Kato Y, Protective role of antioxidative food factors in oxidative stress caused by hyperglycemia. *Ann N Y Acad Sci.* Jun;1043:440-51, 2005

Piconi L, Quagliaro L, Ceriello A., Oxidative stress in diabetes. *Clin Chem Lab Med.* Sep;41(9):1144-9, 2003

Free Radicals, Skin Aging and Cancer

Nishigori C, Hattori Y, Toyokuni S, Role of reactive oxygen species in skin carcinogenesis. *Antioxid Redox Signal.* Jun;6(3):561-70, 2004

Pinnell SR. Cutaneous photodamage, oxidative stress, and topical antioxidant protection. *J Am Acad Dermatol.* Jan;48(1):1-19, 2003

Valencia A, Kochevar IE. Ultraviolet A induces apoptosis via reactive oxygen species in a model for Smith-Lemli-Opitz syndrome. *Free Radic Biol Med.* Feb 15;40(4):641-50, 2006

Free Radical Formation and Cancer

Nowak S, Zukiel R, Barciszewska AM, et al, The diagnosis and therapy of brain tumours. *Folia Neuropathol.* 43(3):193-6, 2005

Petersen DR, Alcohol, iron-associated oxidative stress, and cancer. *Alcohol.* Apr;35(3):243-9, 2005

Poulsen HE, Oxidative DNA modifications. *Exp Toxicol Pathol.* Jul;57 Suppl 1:161-9, 2005

Valko M, Rhodes CJ, Moncol J, et al. Free radicals, metals and antioxidants in oxidative stress-induced cancer. *Chem Biol Interact.* Mar 10;160(1):1-40, 2006

Cooking and Free Radical Formation

Alexander J, Reistad R, Hegstad S, Biomarkers of exposure to heterocyclic amines: approaches to improve the exposure assessment. *Food Chem Toxicol.* Aug;40(8):1131-7, 2002

Banning M.The carcinogenic and protective effects of food. *Br J Nurs.* Nov10-23;14(20):1070-4, 2005

Felton JS, Knize MG, Salmon CP, Human exposure to heterocyclic amine food mutagens/carcinogens: relevance to breast cancer. *Environ Mol Mutagen.* 39(2-3):112-8, 2002

Frederiksen H, Two food-borne heterocyclic amines: metabolism and DNA adduct formation of amino-alpha-carbolines. *Mol Nutr Food Res.* Mar;49(3):263-73, 2005

Knize MG, Felton JS, Formation and human risk of carcinogenic heterocyclic amines formed from natural precursors in meat. *Nutr Rev.* May;63(5):158-65, 2005

Knize MG, Kulp KS, Salmon CP, Factors affecting human heterocyclic amine intake and the metabolism of PhIP. *Mutat Res.* Sep 30;506-507:153-62, 2002

Maeda H, Sato K, Akaike T, Superoxide radical generation from heterocyclic amines. *Princess Takamatsu Symp.* 23:103-12, 1995

Nagao M, A new approach to risk estimation of food-borne carcinogens-heterocyclic amines-based on molecular information. *Mutat Res.* Dec 16;431(1):3-12, 1999

Skog K, Problems associated with the determination of heterocyclic amines in cooked foods and human exposure. *Food Chem Toxicol.* Aug;40(8):1197-203, 2002

Snyderwine EG, Venugopal M, Yu M, Mammary gland carcinogenesis by food-derived heterocyclic amines and studies on the mechanisms of carcinogenesis of 2-amino-1-methyl-6-phenylimidazo[4,5-b]pyridine (PhIP). *Mutat Res.* Sep 30;506-507:145-52, 2002

Sugimura T, Wakabayashi K, Nakagama H, et al, Heterocyclic amines: Mutagens/carcinogens produced during cooking of meat and fish. *Cancer Sci.* Apr;95(4):290-9, 2004

Weisburger JH, Jones RC, Nutritional toxicology: on the mechanisms of inhibition of formation of potent carcinogens during cooking. *Prog Clin Biol Res.* 304:377-90, 1989

Frying and Free Radical Formation

Goburdhun D, Jhaumeer-Laulloo SB, Musruck R, Evaluation of soybean oil quality during conventional frying by FTIR and some chemical indexes. *Int J Food Sci Nutr.* Jan;52(1):31-42, 2001

Paul S, Mittal GS, Regulating the use of degraded oil/fat in deep-fat/oil food frying. *Crit Rev Food Sci Nutr.* Nov;37(7):635-62, 1997

Strickland PT, Qian Z, Friesen MD, Metabolites of 2-amino-1-methyl-6-phenylimidazo(4,5-b)pyridine (PhIP) in human urine after consumption of charbroiled or fried beef. *Mutat Res.* Sep 30;506-507: 163-73, 2002

Skog KI, Johansson MA, Jagerstad MI, Carcinogenic heterocyclic amines in model systems and cooked foods: a review on formation, occurrence and intake. *Food Chem Toxicol.* Sep-Oct;36(9-10):879-96, 1998

Grilling and Free Radical Formation

Grivas S, Synthetic routes to the food carcinogen 2 amino-3,8-dimethylimidazo[4,5-f]quinoxaline (8-MeIQx) and related compounds. *Princess Takamatsu Symp.* 23:1-8, 1995

Sinha R, An epidemiologic approach to studying heterocyclic amines. *Mutat Res.* Sep 30;506-507: 197-204, 2002

Heated Foods and Free Radical Formation

Andlauer W, Stumpf C, Hubert M, et al, Influence of cooking process on phenolic marker compounds of vegetables. *Int J Vitam Nutr Res.* Mar;73(2):152-9, 2003

Silva EM, Simon PW, Genetic, physiological, and environmental factors affecting acrylamide concentration in fried potato products. *Adv Exp Med Biol.* 561:371-86, 2005

Tareke E, Rydberg P, Karlsson P, et al, Analysis of acrylamide, a carcinogen formed in heated foodstuffs. *J Agric Food Chem.* Aug 14;50(17):4998-5006, 2002

Yoshida M, Ono H, Chuda Y, et al, Acrylamide in Japanese processed foods and factors affecting acrylamide level in potato chips and tea. *Adv Exp Med Biol.* 561:405-13, 2005

Yousef MI, El-Demerdash FM, Acrylamide-induced oxidative stress and biochemical perturbations in rats. *Toxicology.* Feb 15;219(1-3):133-41, 2006

Effects of Antioxidants outside the Brain

Brenneisen P, Steinbrenner H, Sies H, Selenium, oxidative stress, and health aspects. *Mol Aspects Med.* Aug-Oct;26(4-5):256-67, 2005

Chainani-Wu N, Diet and oral, pharyngeal, and esophageal cancer. *Nutr Cancer.* 44(2):104-26, 2002

Dryden GW, Song M, McClain C, Polyphenols and gastrointestinal diseases. *Curr Opin Gastroenterol.* Mar;22(2):165-70, 2006

Feskanich D, Ziegler RG, Michaud D, et al, Prospective study of fruit and vegetable consumption and risk of lung cancer among men and women. *J Natl Cancer Inst.* Nov 15;92(22):1812-23, 2000

He FJ, Nowson CA, MacGregor GA, Fruit and vegetable consumption and stroke: meta-analysis of cohort studies. *Lancet.* Jan 28;367(9507):320-6, 2006

Key TJ, Schatzkin A, Willett WC, et al, Diet, nutrition and the prevention of cancer. *Public Health Nutr.* Feb;7(1A):187-200, 2004

La Vecchia C, Mediterranean diet and cancer. *Public Health Nutr.* Oct;7(7):965-8, 2004

La Vecchia C, Altieri A, Tavani A, Vegetables, fruit, antioxidants and cancer: a review of Italian studies. *Eur J Nutr.* Dec;40(6):261-7, 2001

La Vecchia C, Negri E, Nutrition and bladder cancer. *Cancer Causes Control.* Jan;7(1):95-100, 1996

La Vecchia C, Tavani A, Fruit and vegetables, and human cancer. *Eur J Cancer Prev.* Feb;7(1):3-8, 1998

Lawson LD, Gardner CD, Composition, stability, and bioavailability of garlic products used in a clinical trial. *J Agric Food Chem.* Aug 10;53(16):6254-61, 2005

Lewis N, Raud J, Apples and the American diet. *Nutr Clin Care.* Apr-Jun;7(2):82-8, 2004

O'Brien P, Carrasco-Pozo C, Speisky H, Boldine and its antioxidant or health-promoting properties. *Chem Biol Interact.* Oct 10, 2006

Pelucchi C, Talamini R, Negri E, et al, Folate intake and risk of oral and pharyngeal cancer. *Ann Oncol.* Nov;14(11):1677-81, 2003

Ray AL, Semba RD, Walston J, et al, Low serum selenium and total carotenoids predict mortality among older women living in the community: the women's health and aging studies. *J Nutr.* Jan;136(1):172-6, 2006

Rebrin I, Zicker S, Wedekind KJ, et al. Effect of antioxidant-enriched diets on glutathione redox status in tissue homogenates and mitochondria of the senescence-accelerated mouse. *Free Radic Biol Med.* Aug 15;39(4):549-57, 2005

Riboli E, Norat T, Cancer prevention and diet: opportunities in Europe. *Public Health Nutr.* Apr;4(2B):475-84, 2001

Riboli E, Norat T, Epidemiologic evidence of the protective effect of fruit and vegetables on cancer risk. *Am J Clin Nutr.* Sep;78(3 Suppl):559S-569S, 2003

Sen CK, Khanna S, Roy S, Tocotrienols: Vitamin E beyond tocopherols. *Life Sci.* Feb 2, 2006

Tavani A, La Vecchia C, Fruit and vegetable consumption and cancer risk in a Mediterranean population. *Am J Clin Nutr.* Jun;61(6 Suppl):1374S-1377S, 1995

Temple NJ, Gladwin KK, Fruit, vegetables, and the prevention of cancer: research challenges. *Nutrition.* May;19(5):467-70, 2003

Terry P, Terry JB, Wolk A, Fruit and vegetable consumption in the prevention of cancer: an update. *J Intern Med.* Oct;250(4):280-90, 2001

Tucker JM, Townsend DM, Alpha-tocopherol: roles in prevention and therapy of human disease. *Biomed Pharmacother.* Aug;59(7):380-7, 2005

Vinson JA, Al Kharrat H, Andreoli L, Effect of Aloe vera preparations on the human bioavailability of vitamins C and E. *Phytomedicine.* Nov;12(10):760-5, 2005

Young JE, Zhao X, Carey EE, et al, Phytochemical phenolics in organically grown vegetables. *Mol Nutr Food Res.* Dec;49(12):1136-42, 2005

Antioxidants, Cognition and Behavior

Anderson AS, Porteous LE, Foster E, The impact of a school-based nutrition education intervention on dietary intake and cognitive and attitudinal variables relating to fruits and vegetables. *Public Health Nutr.* Sep;8(6):650-6, 2005

Casadesus G, Shukitt-Hale B, Joseph JA., Qualitative versus quantitative caloric intake: are they equivalent paths to successful aging? *Neurobiol Aging.* Sep-Oct;23(5):747-69, 2002

Das A, Shanker G, Nath C, A comparative study in rodents of standardized extracts of Bacopa monniera and Ginkgo biloba: anticholinesterase and cognitive enhancing activities. *Pharmacol Biochem Behav.* Nov;73(4):893-900, 2002

Donahue AN, Aschner M, Lash LH, et al, Growth hormone administration to aged animals reduces disulfide glutathione levels in hippocampus. *Mech Ageing Dev.* 2006 Jan;127(1):57-63. Epub Oct 21, 2005

Fillit HM, Butler RN, O'Connell AW, et al, Achieving and maintaining cognitive vitality with aging. *Mayo Clin Proc.* Jul;77(7):681-96, 2002

Joseph JA, Shukitt-Hale B, Casadesus G, et al, Oxidative stress and inflammation in brain aging: nutritional considerations. *Neurochem Res.* Jun-Jul;30(6-7):927-35, 2005

Joseph JA, Shukitt-Hale B, Casadesus G, Reversing the deleterious effects of aging on brain cellal communication and behavior: beneficial properties of fruit polyphenolic compounds. *Am J Clin Nutr.* Jan;81(1 Suppl):313S-316S, 2005

Joseph JA, Shukitt-Hale B, Denisova NA, et al, Reversals of age-related declines in brain cellal signal transduction, cognitive, and motor behavioral deficits with blueberry, spinach, or strawberry dietary supplementation. *J Neurosci.* Sep 15;19(18):8114-21, 1999

Joseph JA, Shukitt-Hale B, Denisova NA, et al, Long-term dietary strawberry, spinach, or vitamin E supplementation retards the onset of age-related brain cellal signal-transduction and cognitive behavioral deficits. *J Neurosci.* Oct 1;18(19):8047-55, 1998

Kang JH, Ascherio A, Grodstein F, Fruit and vegetable consumption and cognitive decline in aging women. *Ann Neurol.* May;57(5):713-20, 2005

Kidd PM, A review of nutrients and botanicals in the integrative management of cognitive dysfunction. *Altern Med Rev.* Jun;4(3):144-61, 1999

Kolosova NG, Shcheglova TV, Sergeeva SV, et al, Long-term antioxidant supplementation attenuates oxidative stress markers and cognitive deficits in senescent-accelerated OXYS rats. *Neurobiol Aging.* Oct 20, 2005

Lau FC, Shukitt-Hale B, Joseph JA., The beneficial effects of fruit polyphenols on brain aging. *Neurobiol Aging.* Dec;26 Suppl 1:128-32, 2005

Mandel SA, Avramovich-Tirosh Y, Reznichenko L, et al, Multifunctional activities of green tea catechins in neuroprotection. Modulation of cell survival genes, iron-dependent oxidative stress and PKC signaling pathway. *Neurosignals.* 14(1-2):46-60, 2005

Martin A, Cherubini A, Andres-Lacueva C, et al, Effects of fruits and vegetables on levels of vitamins E and C in the brain and their association with cognitive performance. *J Nutr Health Aging.* 6(6):392-404, 2002

Rogers EJ, Milhalik S, Orthiz D, et al, Apple juice prevents oxidative stress and impaired cognitive performance caused by genetic and dietary deficiencies in mice. *J Nutr Health Aging.* 8(2):92-7, 2004

Russo A, Borrelli F, Bacopa monniera, a reputed nootropic plant: an overview. *Phytomedicine.* Apr;12(4):305-17, 2005

Russo A, Borrelli F, Campisi A, et al, Nitric oxide-related toxicity in cultured astrocytes: effect of Bacopa monniera. *Life Sci.* Aug 8;73(12):1517-26, 2003

Russo A, Izzo AA, Borrelli F, et al, Free radical scavenging capacity and protective effect of Bacopa monniera L. on DNA damage. *Phytother Res.* Sep;17(8):870-5, 2003

Sairam K, Dorababu M, Goel RK, et al, Antidepressant activity of standardized extract of Bacopa monniera in experimental models of depression in rats. *Phytomedicine.* Apr;9(3):207-11, 2002

Tucker KL, Stress and nutrition in relation to excess development of chronic disease in Puerto Rican adults living in the Northeastern USA. *J Med Invest.* Nov;52 Suppl:252-8, 2005

Vohora D, Pal SN, Pillai KK, Protection from phenytoin-induced cognitive deficit by Bacopa monniera, a reputed Indian nootropic plant. *J Ethnopharmacol.* Aug;71(3):383-90, 2000

Wu A, Ying Z, Gomez-Pinilla F, Dietary curcumin counteracts the outcome of traumatic brain injury on oxidative stress, synaptic plasticity, and cognition. *Exp Neurol.* Feb;197(2):309-17, 2006

Youdim KA, Spencer JP, Schroeter H, et al. Dietary flavonoids as potential neuroprotectants. *Biol Chem.* Mar-Apr;383(3-4):503-19, 2002

Youdim KA, Shukitt-Hale B, Joseph JA. Flavonoids and the brain: interactions at the blood-brain barrier and their physiological effects on the central nervous system. *Free Radic Biol Med.* Dec 1;37(11):1683-93, 2004

Zicker SC, Cognitive and behavioral assessment in dogs and pet food market applications. *Prog Neuropsychopharmacol Biol Psychiatry.* Mar;29(3):455-9, 2005

Antioxidants and Learning

Abe K, Saito H, Effects of saffron extract and its constituent crocin on learning behaviour and long-term potentiation. *Phytother Res.* May;14(3):149-52, 2000

Contestabile A, Monti B, Contestabile A, et al, Brain nitric oxide and its dual role in neurodegeneration/neuroprotection: understanding molecular mechanisms to devise drug approaches. *Curr Med Chem.* Oct;10(20):2147-74, 2003

Cotman CW, Head E, Muggenburg BA, et al, Brain aging in the canine: a diet enriched in antioxidants reduces cognitive dysfunction. *Neurobiol Aging.* Sep-Oct;23(5):809-18, 2002

Delwing D, Bavaresco CS, Monteiro SC, et al, alpha-Tocopherol and ascorbic acid prevent memory deficits provoked by chronic hyperprolinemia in rats. *Behav Brain Res.* Oct 5; 2005

Gordon N, Newton RW, Glucose transporter type1 (GLUT-1) deficiency. *Brain Dev.* Oct;25(7):477-80, 2003

Head E, Zicker SC, Nutraceuticals, aging, and cognitive dysfunction. *Vet Clin North Am Small Anim Pract.* Jan;34(1):217-28, 2004

Kheirandish L, Row BW, Li RC, et al, Apolipoprotein E-deficient mice exhibit increased vulnerability to intermittent hypoxia-induced spatial learning deficits. *Sleep.* Nov 1;28(11):1412-7, 2005

Maidana M, Carlis V, Galhardi FG, et al, Effects of microcystins over short- and long-term memory and oxidative stress generation in hippocampus of rats. *Chem Biol Interact.* Feb 25;159(3):223-34, 2006

Milgram NW, Head E, Muggenburg B, et al, Landmark discrimination learning in the dog: effects of age, an antioxidant fortified food, and cognitive strategy. *Neurosci Biobehav Rev.* Oct;26(6):679-95, 2002

Mook-Jung I, Hong HS, Boo JH, et al, Ginsenoside Rb1 and Rg1 improve spatial learning and increase hippocampal synaptophysin level in mice. *J Neurosci Res.* Mar 15;63(6):509-15, 2001

Shen YX, Wei W, Yang J, et al, Improvement of melatonin to the learning and memory impairment induced by amyloid beta-peptide 25-35 in elder rats. *Acta Pharmacol Sin.* Sep;22(9):797-803, 2001

Shinomiya K, Tokunaga S, Shigemoto Y, et al, Effect of seed coat extract from black soybeans on radial maze performance in rats. *Clin Exp Pharmacol Physiol.* Sep;32(9):757-60, 2005

Smythies J, The neurochemical basis of learning and neurocomputation: the redox theory. *Behav Brain Res.* Feb 15;99(1):1-6, 1999

Tanaka S, Ide M, Shibutani T, et al, Lipopolysaccharide-induced microglial activation induces learning and memory deficits without brain cellal cell death in rats. *J Neurosci Res.* Jan 20, 2006

Yamada K, Tanaka T, Han D, et al, Protective effects of idebenone and alpha-tocopherol on beta-amyloid-(1-42)-induced learning and memory deficits in rats: implication of oxidative stress in beta-amyloid-induced neurotoxicity in vivo. Eur *J Neurosci.* Jan;11(1):83-90, 1999

Antioxidants and Memory

Andres-Lacueva C, Shukitt-Hale B, Galli RL,et al, Anthocyanins in aged blueberry-fed rats are found centrally and may enhance memory. *Nutr Neurosci.* Apr;8(2):111-20, 2005

Bao HY, Zhang J, Yeo SJ, et al. Memory enhancing and neuroprotective effects of selected ginsenosides. *Arch Pharm Res.* Mar;28(3):335-42, 2005

Ferrari CK. Functional foods, herbs and nutraceuticals: towards biochemical mechanisms of healthy aging. *Biogerontology.* 5(5):275-89, 2004

Galli RL, Shukitt-Hale B, Youdim KA, et al, Fruit polyphenolics and brain aging: nutritional interventions targeting age-related brain cellal and behavioral deficits. *Ann N Y Acad Sci.* Apr;959: 128-32, 2002

Joseph JA, Denisova N, Fisher D, et al, Membrane and receptor modifications of oxidative stress vulnerability in aging. Nutritional considerations. *Ann N Y Acad Sci.* Nov 20;854:268-76, 1998

Lee KY, Jeong EJ, Lee HS, et al, Acteoside of Callicarpa dichotoma attenuates scopolamine-induced memory impairments. *Biol Pharm Bull.* Jan;29(1):71-4, 2006

Levin ED. Extracellular superoxide dismutase (EC-SOD) quenches free radicals and attenuates age-related cognitive decline: opportunities for novel drug development in aging. *Curr Alzheimer Res.* Apr;2(2):191-6, 2005

Mandel S, Packer L, Youdim MB, et al. Proceedings from the "Third International Conference on Mechanism of Action of Nutraceuticals". *J Nutr Biochem.* Sep;16(9):513-20, 2005

Maxwell CJ, Hicks MS, Hogan DB, et al, Supplemental use of antioxidant vitamins and subsequent risk of cognitive decline and dementia. *Dement Geriatr Cogn Disord.* 20(1):45-51, 2005

McDaniel MA, Maier SF, Einstein GO, "Brain-specific" nutrients: a memory cure?. *Nutrition.* Nov-Dec;19(11-12):957-75, 2003

Miller DB, O'Callaghan JP, Aging, stress and the hippocampus. *Ageing Res Rev.* May;4(2):123-40, 2005

Miller JW, Vitamin E and memory: is it vascular protection? *Nutr Rev.* Apr;58(4):109-11, 2000

Perrig WJ, Perrig P, Stahelin HB, The relation between antioxidants and memory performance in the old and very old, *J Am Geriatr Soc.* Jun;45(6):718-24, 1997

Ramirez MR, Izquierdo I, do Carmo Bassols Raseira M, et al, Effect of lyophilised Vaccinium berries on memory, anxiety and locomotion in adult rats. *Pharmacol Res.* Dec;52(6):457-62, 2005

Tabet N, Mantle D, Walker Z, et al, Higher fat and carbohydrate intake in dementia patients is associated with increased blood glutathione peroxidase activity. *Int Psychogeriatr.* Mar;17(1):91-8, 2005

Youdim KA, Joseph JA, A possible emerging role of phytochemicals in improving age-related neurological dysfunctions: a multiplicity of effects. *Free Radic Biol Med.* Mar 15;30(6):583-94, 2001

Antioxidants and Mild Cognitive Impairment

Berr C, Oxidative stress and cognitive impairment in the elderly. *J Nutr Health Aging.* 6(4):261-6, 2002

Deschamps V, Barberger-Gateau P, et al, Nutritional factors in cerebral aging and dementia: epidemiological arguments for a role of oxidative stress. *Neuroepidemiology.* Feb;20(1):7-15, 2001

Jelic V, Winblad B, Treatment of mild cognitive impairment: rationale, present and future strategies. *Acta Neurol Scand Suppl.* 179:83-93, 2003

Joseph JA, Denisova NA, Bielinski D, et al, Oxidative stress protection and vulnerability in aging: putative nutritional implications for intervention. *Mech Ageing Dev.* Jul 31;116(2-3):141-53, 2000

Mecocci P. Oxidative stress in mild cognitive impairment and Alzheimer disease: a continuum. *J Alzheimers Dis.* Apr;6(2):159-63, 2004

Mecocci P, Mariani E, Cornacchiola V, et al. Antioxidants for the treatment of mild cognitive impairment. *Neurol Res.* Jul;26(5):598-602, 2004

Petersen RC, Thomas RG, Grundman M, et al, Vitamin E and donepezil for the treatment of mild cognitive impairment. *N Engl J Med.* Jun 9;352(23):2379-88, 2005

Pratico D, Clark CM, Liun F, et al, Increase of brain oxidative stress in mild cognitive impairment: a possible predictor of Alzheimer disease. *Arch Neurol.* Sep;59(9):1475, 2002

Quinn JF, Bussiere JR, Hammond RS, et al. Chronic dietary alpha-lipoic acid reduces deficits in hippocampal memory of aged Tg2576 mice. *Neurobiol Aging.* Jan 28, 2006

Rinaldi P, Polidori MC, Metastasio A, et al. Plasma antioxidants are similarly depleted in mild cognitive impairment and in Alzheimer's disease. *Neurobiol Aging.* Nov;24(7):915-9, 2003

Voisin T, Touchon J, Vellas B, Mild cognitive impairment: a nosological entity? *Curr Opin Neurol.* Dec;16 Suppl 2:S43-5, 2003

Antioxidants, Alzheimer's and Other Neurodegenerative Diseases

Aliev G, Smith MA, Obrenovich ME, et al, Role of vascular hypoperfusion-induced oxidative stress and mitochondria failure in the pathogenesis of Azheimer disease. *Neurotox Res.* 5(7):491-504, 2003

Behl C, Oxidative stress in Alzheimer's disease: implications for prevention and therapy. Subcell Biochem. 38:65-78, 2005

Butterfield DA, Castegna A, Drake J, et al, Vitamin E and neurodegenerative disorders associated with oxidative stress. *Nutr Neurosci.* Sep;5(4):229-39, 2002

Gahtan E, Overmier JB, Inflammatory pathogenesis in Alzheimer's disease: biological mechanisms and cognitive sequeli. *Neurosci Biobehav Rev.* May;23(5):615-33, 1999

Gilgun-Sherki Y, Melamed E, Offen D, Antioxidant treatment in Alzheimer's disease: current state. *J Mol Neurosci.* 21(1):1-11, 2003

Grundman M, Vitamin E and Alzheimer disease: the basis for additional clinical trials. *Am J Clin Nutr.* Feb;71(2):630S-636S, 2000

Grundman M, Grundman M, Delaney P. Antioxidant strategies for Alzheimer's disease. *Proc Nutr Soc.* May;61(2):191-202, 2002

Mattson MP, Pedersen WA, Duan W, et al. Cellular and molecular mechanisms underlying perturbed energy metabolism and brain cellal degeneration in Alzheimer's and Parkinson's diseases. *Ann N Y Acad Sci.* 893:154-75, 1999

Pereira C, Agostinho P, Moreira PI, et al, Alzheimer's disease-associated neurotoxic mechanisms and neuroprotective strategies. *Curr Drug Targets CNS Neurol Disord.* Aug;4(4):383-403, 2005

Rao AV, Balachandran B, Role of oxidative stress and antioxidants in neurodegenerative diseases. *Nutr Neurosci.* Oct;5(5):291-309, 2002

Rutten BP, Steinbusch HW, Korr H, et al, Antioxidants and Alzheimer's disease: from bench to bedside (and back again). *Curr Opin Clin Nutr Metab Care.* Nov;5(6):645-51, 2002

Souder E, Neuropathology in Alzheimer's disease: target of pharmacotherapy. *J Am Acad Nurse Pract.* Mar; Suppl:3-5, 2005

Vina J, Lloret A, Orti R, et al, Molecular bases of the treatment of Alzheimer's disease with antioxidants: prevention of oxidative stress. *Mol Aspects Med.* Feb-Apr;25(1-2):117-23, 2004

Yan JJ, Cho JY, Kim HS, et al. Protection against beta-amyloid peptide toxicity in vivo with long-term administration of ferulic acid. *Br J Pharmacol.* May;133(1):89-96, 2001

Bioavailability of Brand versus Generic Prescription Medicines

Borgheini G, The bioequivalence and therapeutic efficacy of generic versus brand-name psychoactive drugs. *Clin Ther.* Jun;25(6):1578-92, 2003

Burkhardt RT, Leppik IE, Scott S, et al, Lower phenytoin serum levels in persons switched from brand to generic phenytoin. *Neurology.* Oct 26;63(8):1494-6, 2004

Diamond BI, Albrecht JW, Drug substitution in transplantation: a National Kidney Foundation White Paper. *Psychopathology.* 20 Suppl 1:92-8, 1987

Henderson JD, Esham RH, Generic substitution: issues for problematic drugs. *South Med J.* Jan;94(1):16-21, 2001

Reiffel JA, Issues in the use of generic antiarrhythmic drugs. *Curr opin Cardiol.* Jan;16(1):23-9, 2001

Sabatini S, Ferguson RM, Helderman JH, et al, Drug substitution in transplantation: a National Kidney Foundation White Paper. *Am J Kidney Dis.* Feb;33(2):389-97, 1999

Tse G, Thompson D, Procyshyn RM, Generic clozapine: a cost-saving alternative to brand name clozapine? *Pharmacoeconomics.* 21(1):1-11, 2003

Bluberries Are Good but No Great Shakes

Kurilich AC, Clevidence BA, Britz SJ, et al, Plasma and urine responses are lower for acylated vs nonacylated anthocyanins from raw and cooked purple carrots. *J Agric Food Chem.* Aug 10;53(16):6537-42, 2005

McDougall GJ, Fyffe S, Dobson P, Anthocyanins from red wine-their stability under simulated gastrointestinal digestion. *Phytochemistry.* Nov;66(21):2540-8, 2005

Prior RL, Fruits and vegetables in the prevention of cellular oxidative damage. *Am J Clin Nutr.* Sep; 78(3 Suppl):570S-578S, 2003

Prior RL, Cao G, Prior RL, et al, Analysis of botanicals and dietary supplements for antioxidant capacity: a review. *J AOAC Int.* Jul-Aug;83(4):950-6, 2000

Szeto YT, Tomlinson B, Benzie IF, Total antioxidant and ascorbic acid content of fresh fruits and vegetables: implications for dietary planning and food preservation. *Br J Nutr.* Jan;87(1):55-9, 2002

van der Gaag MS, van den Berg R, van den Berg H, et al. Moderate consumption of beer, red wine and spirits has counteracting effects on plasma antioxidants in middle-aged men. *Eur J Clin Nutr.* Jul;54(7):586-91, 2000

Wu X, Pittman HE 3rd, Prior RL, Fate of anthocyanins and antioxidant capacity in contents of the gastrointestinal tract of weanling pigs following black raspberry consumption. *J Agric Food Chem.* Jan 25;54(2):583-9, 2006

Popeye Could Have Been Even Smarter

Pandjaitan N, Howard LR, Morelock T, et al, Antioxidant capacity and phenolic content of spinach as affected by genetics and maturation. *J Agric Food Chem.* Nov 2;53(22):8618-23, 2005

Riso P, Brusamolino A, Scalfi L, et al, Bioavailability of carotenoids from spinach and tomatoes. *Nutr Metab Cardiovasc Dis.* Jun;14(3):150-6, 2004

Tang G, Qin J, Dolnikowski GG, et al, Spinach or carrots can supply significant amounts of vitamin A as assessed by feeding with intrinsically deuterated vegetables. *Am J Clin Nutr.* Oct;82(4):821-8, 2005

Empty Waves of Grain

Adom KK, Sorrells ME, Liu RH, Phytochemicals and antioxidant activity of milled fractions of different wheat varieties. *J Agric Food Chem.* Mar 23;53(6):2297-306, 2005

Baublis AJ, Lu C, Clydesdale FM, et al, Potential of wheat-based breakfast cereals as a source of dietary antioxidants. *J Am Coll Nutr.* Jun;19(3 Suppl):308S-311S, 2000

Bingham SA, Norat T, Moskal A, et al, Is the association with fiber from foods in colorectal cancer confounded by folate intake? *Cancer Epidemiol Biomarkers Prev.* Jun;14(6):1552-6, 2005.

Mpofu A, Sapirstein HD, Beta T, Genotype and environmental variation in phenolic content, phenolic acid composition, and antioxidant activity of hard spring wheat. *J Agric Food Chem.* Feb 22;54(4):1265-70, 2006

Shaw CA, Bains JS, Did consumption of flour bleached by the agene process contribute to the incidence of neurological disease? *Med Hypotheses.* Dec;51(6):477-81, 1998

Iced Tea Rules When Made Fresh

Fujiki H, Suganuma M, Imai K, et al, Green tea: cancer preventive beverage and/or drug. *Cancer Lett.* Dec 15;188(1-2):9-13, 2002

Frei B, Higdon JV, Antioxidant activity of tea polyphenols in vivo: evidence from animal studies. *J Nutr.* Oct;133(10):3275S-84S, 2003

Henning SM, Fajardo-Lira C, Lee HW, Catechin content of 18 teas and a green tea extract supplement correlates with the antioxidant capacity. *Nutr Cancer.* 45(2):226-35, 2003

Henning SM, Niu Y, Lee NH, et al, Bioavailability and antioxidant activity of tea flavanols after consumption of green tea, black tea, or a green tea extract supplement. *Am J Clin Nutr.* Dec;80(6):1558-64, 2004

Higdon JV, Frei B, Tea catechins and polyphenols: health effects, metabolism, and antioxidant functions. *Crit Rev Food Sci Nutr.* 43(1):89-143, 2003

Leung LK, Su Y, Chen R, et al, Theaflavins in black tea and catechins in green tea are equally effective antioxidants. *J Nutr.* Sep;131(9):2248-51, 2001

Luczaj W, Skrzydlewska E, Antioxidative properties of black tea. *Prev Med.* Jun;40(6):910-8, 2005

Prior RL, Cao G, In vivo total antioxidant capacity: comparison of different analytical methods. *Free Radic Biol Med.* Dec;27(11-12):1173-81, 1999

Prior RL, Cao G, Antioxidant capacity and polyphenolic components of teas: implications for altering in vivo antioxidant status. *Proc Soc Exp Biol Med.* Apr;220(4):255-61, 1999

Richelle M, Tavazzi I, Offord E, Comparison of the antioxidant activity of commonly consumed polyphenolic beverages (coffee, cocoa, and tea) prepared per cup serving. *J Agric Food Chem.* Jul;49(7):3438-42, 2001

Schmidt M, Schmitz HJ, Baumgart A, Toxicity of green tea extracts and their constituents in rat hepatocytes in primary culture. *Food Chem Toxicol.* Feb;43(2):307-14, 2005

Terao J, Dietary flavonoids as antioxidants in vivo: conjugated metabolites of (-)-epicatechin and quercetin participate in antioxidative defense in blood plasma. *J Med Invest.* Aug;46(3-4):159-68, 1999

Williamson G, Manach C, Bioavailability and bioefficacy of polyphenols in humans. II. Review of 93 intervention studies. *Am J Clin Nutr.* Jan;81(1 Suppl):243S-255S, 2005

Lycopene Loves Processing

Bohm V, Bitsch R, Intestinal absorption of lycopene from different matrices and interactions to other carotenoids, the lipid status, and the antioxidant capacity of human plasma. Eur *J Nutr.* Jun;38(3):118-25, 1999

Caris-Veyrat C, Amiot MJ, Tyssandier V, et al, Influence of organic versus conventional agricultural practice on the antioxidant microconstituent content of tomatoes and derived purees; consequences on antioxidant plasma status in humans. *J Agric Food Chem.* Oct 20;52(21):6503-9, 2004

Cohn W, Thurmann P, Tenter U, et al, Comparative multiple dose plasma kinetics of lycopene administered in tomato juice, tomato soup or lycopene tablets. Eur *J Nutr.* Oct;43(5):304-12, 2004

Paetau I, Khachik F, Brown ED, Chronic ingestion of lycopene-rich tomato juice or lycopene supplements significantly increases plasma concentrations of lycopene and related tomato carotenoids in humans. *Am J Clin Nutr.* Dec;68(6):1187-95, 1998

What Good Are Vital Oils?

Alarcon de la Lastra C, Barranco MD, Motilva V, et al, Mediterranean diet and health: biological importance of olive oil. *Curr Pharm Des.* Jul;7(10):933-50, 2001

Berry EM, Dietary fatty acids in the management of diabetes mellitus. *Am J Clin Nutr.* Oct;66(4 Suppl):991S-997S, 1997

Corrocher R, Pagnan A, Ambrosio GB, et al, Effects induced by olive oil-rich diet on erythrocytes membrane lipids and sodium-potassium transports in postmenopausal hypertensive women. *J Endocrinol Invest.* May;15(5):369-76, 1992

Hashim YZ, Eng M, Gill CI, et al. Components of olive oil and chemoprevention of colorectal cancer. *Nutr Rev.* Nov;63(11):374-86, 2005

Heyden S, Polyunsaturated and monounsaturated fatty acids in the diet to prevent coronary heart disease via cholesterol reduction. *Ann Nutr Metab.* 38(3):117-22, 1994

Manthey FA, Lee RE, Hall CA 3rd, Processing and cooking effects on lipid content and stability of alpha-linolenic acid in spaghetti containing ground flaxseed. *J Agric Food Chem.* Mar 13;50(6):1668-7, 2002

Owen RW, Haubner R, Wurtele G, et al, Olives and olive oil in cancer prevention. *Eur J Cancer Prev.* Aug;13(4):319-26, 2004

Paul S, Mittal GS, Regulating the use of degraded oil/fat in deep-fat/oil food frying. *Crit Rev Food Sci Nutr.* Nov;37(7):635-62, 1997

Perona JS, Cabello-Moruno R, Ruiz-Gutierrez V, The role of virgin olive oil components in the modulation of endothelial function. *J Nutr Biochem.* Dec 12, 2005

Wanasundara PK, Shahidi F, Process-induced compositional changes of flaxseed. *Adv Exp Med Biol.* 434:307-25, 1998

Vital Oils, Brain Cells and the Mind

Agostoni C, Giovannini M, Cognitive and visual development: influence of differences in breast and formula fed infants. *Nutr Health.* 15(3-4):183-8, 2001

Alessandri JM, Goustard B, Guesnet P, et al, Docosahexaenoic acid concentrations in retinal phospholipids of piglets fed an infant formula enriched with long-chain polyunsaturated fatty acids: effects of egg phospholipids and fish oils with different ratios of eicosapentaenoic acid to docosahexaenoic acid. *Am J Clin Nutr.* Mar;67(3):377-85, 1998

Alessandri JM, Guesnet P, Vancassel S, et al, Polyunsaturated fatty acids in the central nervous system: evolution of concepts and nutritional implications throughout life. *Reprod Nutr Dev.* Nov-Dec;44(6):509-38, 2004

Arlt S, Beisiegel U, Kontush A, Lipid peroxidation in neurodegeneration: new insights into Alzheimer's disease. *Curr Opin Lipidol.* Jun;13(3):289-94, 2002

Auestad N, Scott DT, Janowsky JS, et al, Visual, cognitive, and language assessments at 39 months: a follow-up study of children fed formulas containing long-chain polyunsaturated fatty acids to 1 year of age. *Pediatrics.* Sep;112(3 Pt 1):e177-83, 2003

Bassett CN, Montine TJ, Lipoproteins and lipid peroxidation in Alzheimer's disease. *J Nutr Health Aging.* 7(1):24-9, 2003

Bazan NG, Synaptic lipid signaling: significance of polyunsaturated fatty acids and platelet-activating factor. *J Lipid Res.* Dec;44(12):2221-33, 2003

Bourre JM, Roles of unsaturated fatty acids (especially omega-3 fatty acids) in the brain at various ages and during ageing. *J Nutr Health Aging.* 8(3):163-74, 2004

Bourre JM, Free radicals, polyunsaturated fatty acids, cell death, brain aging. *C R Seances Soc Biol Fil.* 182(1):5-36, 1988

Burdge GC, Calder PC, Conversion of alpha-linolenic acid to longer-chain polyunsaturated fatty acids in human adults. *Reprod Nutr Dev.* Sep-Oct;45(5):581-97, 2005

Burgess JR, Stevens L, Zhang W, et al. Long-chain polyunsaturated fatty acids in children with attention-deficit hyperactivity disorder. *Am J Clin Nutr.* Jan;71(1 Suppl):327S-30S, 2000

Carlson SE, Behavioral methods used in the study of long-chain polyunsaturated fatty acid nutrition in primate infants. *Am J Clin Nutr.* Jan;71(1 Suppl):268S-74S, 2000

Chen C, Bazan NG. Lipid signaling: sleep, synaptic plasticity, and neuroprotection. *Prostaglandins Other Lipid Mediat.* Sep;77(1-4):65-76, 2005

Colin A, Reggers J, Castronovo , et al, Lipids, depression and suicide. *Encephale.* Jan-Feb;29(1):49-58, 2003

Colombo J, Recent advances in infant cognition: implications for long-chain polyunsaturated fatty acid supplementation studies. *Lipids.* Sep;36(9):919-26, 2001

Combrinck M, Williams J, De Berardinis MA, et al, Levels of CSF prostaglandin E2, cognitive decline, and survival in Alzheimer's disease. *J Neurol Neurosurg Psychiatry.* Jan;77(1):85-8, 2006

Das UN, Can perinatal supplementation of long-chain polyunsaturated fatty acids prevents schizophrenia in adult life? *Med Sci Monit.* Dec;10(12):HY33-7, 2004

Farkas E, de Wilde MC, Kiliaan AJ, et al, Chronic cerebral hypoperfusion-related neuropathologic changes and compromised cognitive status: window of treatment. *Drugs Today (Barc).* May;38(5):365-76, 2002

Filburn CR, Griffin D, Canine plasma and erythrocyte response to a docosahexaenoic acid-enriched supplement: characterization and potential benefits. *Vet Ther.* Spring;6(1):29-42, 2005

Fioravanti M, Yanagi M, Cytidinediphosphocholine (CDP-choline) for cognitive and behavioural disturbances associated with chronic cerebral disorders in the elderly. *Cochrane Database Syst Rev.* Apr 18;(2):CD000269, 2005

Fleith M, Clandinin MT, Dietary PUFA for preterm and term infants: review of clinical studies. *Crit Rev Food Sci Nutr.* 45(3):205-29, 2005

Fontani G, Corradeschi F, Felici A, et al, Cognitive and physiological effects of Omega-3 polyunsaturated fatty acid supplementation in healthy subjects. *Eur J Clin Invest.* Nov;35(11):691-9, 2005

Garcia-Calatayud S, Redondo C, Martin E, et al, Brain docosahexaenoic acid status and learning in young rats submitted to dietary long-chain polyunsaturated fatty acid deficiency and supplementation limited to lactation. *Pediatr Res.* May;57(5 Pt 1):719-23, 2005

Green P, Yavin E, Mechanisms of docosahexaenoic acid accretion in the fetal brain. *J Neurosci Res.* Apr 15;52(2):129-36, 1998

Gur RC, Brain maturation and its relevance to understanding criminal culpability of juveniles. *Curr Psychiatry Rep.* Aug;7(4):292-6, 2005

Hadders-Algra M, The role of long-chain polyunsaturated fatty acids (LCPUFA) in growth and development. *Adv Exp Med Biol.* 569:80-94, 2005

Heird WC, Lapillonne A, The role of essential fatty acids in development. *Annu Rev Nutr.* 25:549-71, 2005

Heyden S, Polyunsaturated and monounsaturated fatty acids in the diet to prevent coronary heart disease via cholesterol reduction. *Ann Nutr Metab.* 38(3):117-22, 1994

Horrocks LA, Farooqui AA, Docosahexaenoic acid in the diet: its importance in maintenance and restoration of neural membrane function. *Prostaglandins Leukot Essent Fatty Acids.* Apr;70(4):361-72, 2004

Innis SM, Perinatal biochemistry and physiology of long-chain polyunsaturated fatty acids. *J Pediatr.* Oct;143(4 Suppl):S1-8, 2003

Itomura M, Hamazaki K, Sawazaki S, et al, The effect of fish oil on physical aggression in school children-a randomized, double-blind, placebo-controlled trial. *J Nutr Biochem.* Mar;16(3):163-71, 2005

Joshi K, Lad S, Kale M, et al, Supplementation with flax oil and vitamin C improves the outcome of Attention Deficit Hyperactivity Disorder (ADHD). *Prostaglandins Leukot Essent Fatty Acids.* Jan;74(1):17-21, 2006

Kaplan RJ, Greenwood CE, Dietary saturated fatty acids and brain function. *Neurochem Res.* May;23(5):615-26, 1998

Lefkowitz W, Lim SY, Lin Y, et al, Where does the developing brain obtain its docosahexaenoic acid? Relative contributions of dietary alpha-linolenic acid, docosahexaenoic acid, and body stores in the developing rat. *Pediatr Res.* Jan;57(1):157-65, 2005

Lim SY, Hoshiba J, Salem N Jr, An extraordinary degree of structural specificity is required in neural phospholipids for optimal brain function: n-6 docosapentaenoic acid substitution for docosahexaenoic acid leads to a loss in spatial task performance. *J Neurochem.* Nov;95(3):848-57, 2005

McCann JC, Ames BN, Is docosahexaenoic acid, an n-3 long-chain polyunsaturated fatty acid, required for development of normal brain function? An overview of evidence from cognitive and behavioral tests in humans and animals. *Am J Clin Nutr.* Aug;82(2):281-95, 2005

Mitchell EA, Aman MG, Turbott SH, et al. Clinical characteristics and serum essential fatty acid levels in hyperactive children. *Clin Pediatr (Phila).* Aug;26(8):406-11, 1987

Montine TJ, Montine KS, McMahan W, et al, F2-isoprostanes in Alzheimer and other neurodegenerative diseases. *Antioxid Redox Signal.* Jan-Feb;7(1-2):269-75, 2005

Montine TJ, Morrow JD, Fatty acid oxidation in the pathogenesis of Alzheimer's disease. *Am J Pathol.* May;166(5):1283-9, 2005

Montine TJ, Neely MD, Quinn JF, et al, Lipid peroxidation in aging brain and Alzheimer's disease. *Free Radic Biol Med.* Sep 1;33(5):620-6, 2002

Montine KS, Quinn JF, Zhang J, et al, Isoprostanes and related products of lipid peroxidation in neurodegenerative diseases. *Chem Phys Lipids.* Mar;128(1-2):117-24, 2004

Moriguchi T, Salem N Jr, Recovery of brain docosahexaenoate leads to recovery of spatial task performance. *J Neurochem.* Oct;87(2):297-309, 2003

Owen RW, Giacosa A, Hull WE, et al, Olive-oil consumption and health: the possible role of antioxidants. *Lancet Oncol.* Oct;1:107-12, 2000

Park YS, Jang HJ, Lee KH, et al, Prolyl endopeptidase inhibitory activity of unsaturated fatty acids. *J Agric Food Chem.* Feb 22;54(4):1238-42, 2006

Perez-Jimenez F, International conference on the healthy effect of virgin olive oil. *Eur J Clin Invest.* Jul;35(7):421-4, 2005

Quinn JF, Bussiere JR, Hammond RS, et al. Chronic dietary alpha-lipoic acid reduces deficits in hippocampal memory of aged Tg2576 mice. *Neurobiol Aging.* Jan 28, 2006

Richardson AJ, Long-chain polyunsaturated fatty acids in childhood developmental and psychiatric disorders. *Lipids.* Dec;39(12):1215-22, 2004

Richardso AJ, Puri BK, A randomized double-blind, placebo-controlled study of the effects of supplementation with highly unsaturated fatty acids on ADHD-related symptoms in children with specific learning difficulties. *Prog Neuropsychopharmacol Biol Psychiatry.* Feb;26(2):233-9, 2002

Riva E, Verduci E, Agostoni C, Closer to the gold standard: an appraisal of formulae available in Italy for use in formula-fed infants. *J Int Med Res.* Nov-Dec;33(6):595-611, 2005

Singh RB, Pella D, Mechirova V, et al, Can brain dysfunction be a predisposing factor for metabolic syndrome? *Biomed Pharmacother.* Oct;58 Suppl 1:S56-68, 2004

Solfrizzi V, D'Introno A, Colacicco AM, et al, Dietary fatty acids intake: possible role in cognitive decline and dementia. *Exp Gerontol.* Apr;40(4):257-70, 2005

Stevens L, Zhang W, Peck L, et al. EFA supplementation in children with inattention, hyperactivity, and other disruptive behaviors. *Lipids.* Oct;38(10):1007-21, 2003

Stillwell W, Shaikh SR, Zerouga M, et al, Docosahexaenoic acid affects cell signaling by altering lipid rafts. *Reprod Nutr Dev.* Sep-Oct;45(5):559-79, 2005

Uauy R, Hoffman DR, Mena P, et al, Term infant studies of DHA and ARA supplementation on neurodevelopment: results of randomized controlled trials. *J Pediatr.* Oct;143(4 Suppl):S17-25, 2003

Valk EE, Hornstra G, Relationship between vitamin E requirement and polyunsaturated fatty acid intake in man: a review. *Int J Vitam Nutr Res.* Mar;70(2):31-42, 2000

Wainwright PE, Dietary essential fatty acids and brain function: a developmental perspective on mechanisms. *Proc Nutr Soc.* Feb;61(1):61-9, 2002

Willatts P, Forsyth JS, The role of long-chain polyunsaturated fatty acids in infant cognitive development. *Prostaglandins Leukot Essent Fatty Acids.* Jul-Aug;63(1-2):95-100, 2000

Yao Y, Clark CM, Trojanowski JQ, et al, Elevation of 12/15 lipoxygenase products in AD and mild cognitive impairment. *Ann Neurol.* Oct;58(4):623-6, 2005

Yehuda S, Rabinovitz S, Carasso RL, et al. The role of polyunsaturated fatty acids in restoring the aging brain cellal membrane. *Neurobiol Aging.* Sep-Oct;23(5):843-53, 2002

Young GS, Conquer JA, Thomas R, Effect of randomized supplementation with high dose olive, flax or fish oil on serum phospholipid fatty acid levels in adults with attention deficit hyperactivity disorder. *Reprod Nutr Dev.* Sep-Oct;45(5):549-58, 2005

The Right Ratio Yields the Right Results

Basu A, Devaraj S, Jialal I, Dietary Factors That Promote or Retard Inflammation. *Arterioscler Thromb Vasc Biol.* Feb 16, 2006

Bezard J, Blond JP, Bernard A, et al, The metabolism and availability of essential fatty acids in animal and human tissues. *Reprod Nutr Dev.* 34(6):539-68, 1994

Broughton KS, Wade JW, Total fat and (n-3)(n-6) fat ratios influence eicosanoid production in mice. *J Nutr.* Jan;132(1):88-94, 2002

Canada Health and Welfare, Health Protection Branch, Bureau of Nutritional Services. *1990 Nutrition Recommendations.* Ottowa, 1990

Collett ED, Davidson LA, Fan YY, et al, n-6 and n-3 polyunsaturated fatty acids differentially modulate oncogenic Ras activation in colonocytes. *Am J Physiol Cell Physiol.* May;280(5):C1066-75, 2001

de Jonge HW, Dekkers DH, Lamers JM, Polyunsaturated fatty acids and signalling via phospholipase C-beta and A2 in myocardium. *Mol Cell Biochem.* Apr 12-26;157(1-2):199-210, 1996

Delarue J, LeFoll C, Corporeau C, et al, N-3 long chain polyunsaturated fatty acids: a nutritional tool to prevent insulin resistance associated to type 2 diabetes and obesity? *Reprod Nutr Dev.* May-Jun;44(3):289-99, 2004

Galella G, Marangoni F, Rise P, et al, n-6 and n-3 fatty acid accumulation in thp-1 cell phospholipids. *Biochim Biophys Acta.* Sep 8;1169(3):280-90, 1993

Gali C, Marangoni F, Recent advances in the biology of n-6 fatty acids. *Nutrition.* Nov-Dec;13(11-12):978-85, 1997

Galli C, Marangoni F, Galella, Modulation of lipid derived mediators by polyunsaturated fatty acids. *Prostaglandins Leukot Essent Fatty Acids.* Jan;48(1):51-5, 1993

Gibson RA, Makrides M, Neumann MA, et al, Ratios of linoleic acid to alpha-linolenic acid in formulas for term infants. *J Pediatr.* Nov;125(5 Pt 2):S48-55, 1994

Harbige LS, Fatty acids, the immune response, and autoimmunity: a question of n-6 essentiality and the balance between n-6 and n-3. *Lipids.* Apr;38(4):323-41, 2003

Koletzko B, Agostoni C, Carlson SE, et al, Long chain polyunsaturated fatty acids (LC-PUFA) and perinatal development. *Acta Paediatr.* Apr;90(4):460-4, 2001

Koo WW, Efficacy and safety of docosahexaenoic acid and arachidonic acid addition to infant formulas: can one buy better vision and intelligence? *J Am Coll Nutr.* Apr;22(2):101-7, 2003

Lands WE, Biochemistry and physiology of n-3 fatty acids. *FASEB J.* May;6(8):2530-6, 1992

Lewis NM, Seburg S, Flanagan NL, Enriched eggs as a source of n-3 polyunsaturated fatty acids for human. *Poult Sci.* Jul;79(7):971-4, 2000

Lindskog M, Gleissman H, Ponthan F, et al, Neuroblastoma cell death in response to docosahexaenoic acid: Sensitization to chemotherapy and arsenic-induced oxidative stress. *Int J Cancer.* Dec 13;118(10):2584-2593, 2005

Navarro MD, Periago JL, Pita ML, et al, The n-3 polyunsaturated fatty acid levels in rat tissue lipids increase in response to dietary olive oil relative to sunflower oil. *Lipids.* Dec;29(12):845-9, 1994

Niki E, Yoshida Y, Saito Y, et al. Lipid peroxidation: mechanisms, inhibition, and biological effects. *Biochem Biophys Res Commun.* Dec 9;338(1):668-76, 2005

Owen RW, Giacosa A, Hull WE, et al, Olive-oil consumption and health: the possible role of antioxidants. *Lancet Oncol.* Oct;1:107-12, 2000

Ozkan Y, Yilmaz O, Ozturk AI, et al, Effects of triple antioxidant combination (vitamin E, vitamin C and alpha-lipoic acid) with insulin on lipid and cholesterol levels and fatty acid composition of brain tissue in experimental diabetic and non-diabetic rats. *Cell Biol Int.* Sep;29(9):754-60, 2005

Renaud S, Lanzmann-Petithory D, Coronary heart disease: dietary links and pathogenesis. *Public Health Nutr.* Apr;4(2B):459-74, 2001

Ruiz-Gutierrez V, Muriana FJ, et al, Plasma lipids, erythrocyte membrane lipids and blood pressure of hypertensive women after ingestion of dietary oleic acid from two different sources. *J Hypertens.* Dec;14(12):1483-90, 1996

Sanigorski AJ, Sinclair, Hamazaki T, Platelet and aorta arachidonic and eicosapentaenoic acid levels and in vitro eicosanoid production in rats fed high-fat diets. *Lipids.* Jul;31(7):729-35, 1996

Sardesai VM, The essential fatty acids. *Nutr Clin Pract.* Aug;7(4):179-86, 1992

Sinopoulos AP, Human requirement for N-3 polyunsaturated fatty acids. *Poult Sci.* Jul;79(7):961-70, 2000

Thies F, Nebe-von-Caron G, Powell JR, et al, Dietary supplementation with eicosapentaenoic acid, but not with other long-chain n-3 or n-6 polyunsaturated fatty acids, drcreases natural killer cell activity in healthy subjects aged >55 y. *Am J Clin Nutr.* Mar;73(3):539-48, 2001

Visioli F, Galli C, Antiatherogenic components of olive oil. *Curr Atheroscler Rep.* Jan;3(1):64-7, 2001

Wahle KW, Caruso D, Ochoa JJ, et al, Olive oil and modulation of cell signaling in disease prevention. *Lipids.* Dec;39(12):1223-31, 2004

Wander RC, Hall JA, Grandin JL, et al, The ratio of dietary (n-6) to (n-3) fatty acids influences immune system function, eicosanoid metabolism, lipid peroxidation and vitamin E status in aged dogs. *J Nutr.* June;127(6):1198-205, 1997

Yaqoob P, Monounsaturated fatty acids and immune function. *Eur J Clin Nutr.* Aug;56 Suppl 3:S9-S13, 2002

We're All Pisces in One Way

Cunnane SC, The Canadian Society for Nutritional Sciences 1995 Young Scientist Award Lecture. Recent studies on the synthesis, beta-oxidation, and deficiency of linoleate and alpha-linolenate: are essential fatty acids more aptly named indispensable or conditionally dispensable fatty acids? *Can J Physiol Pharmacol.* Jun;74(6):629-39, 1996

Cunnane SC, Application of new methods and analytical approaches to research on polyunsaturated fatty acid homeostasis. *Lipids.* Sep;36(9):975-9, 2001

Cunnane SC, Problems with essential fatty acids: time for a new paradigm? *Prog Lipid Res.* Nov;42(6):544-68, 2003

Cunnane SC, Nadeau CR, Likhodii SS, NMR and isotope ratio mass spectrometry studies of in vivo uptake and metabolism of polyunsaturates by the developing rat brain. *J Mol Neurosci.* Apr-Jun;16(2-3):173-80, 2001

Cunnane SC, Ross R, Bannister JL, et al, Beta-oxidation of linoleate in obese men undergoing weight loss. *Am J Clin Nutr.* Apr;73(4):709-14, 2001

Cunnane SC, Ryan MA, Craig KS, et al, Synthesis of linoleate and alpha-linoleate by chain elongation in the rat. *Lipids.* Aug;30(8): 781-3, 1995

Cunnane SC, Ryan MA, Lin YH, et al, Suckling rats actively recycle carbon from alpha-linolenate into newly synthesized lipids even during extreme dietary deficiency of n-3 polyunsaturates. *Pediatr Res.* Jan;59(1):107-10, 2006

Cunnane SC, Ryan MA, Nadeau CR, et al, Why is carbon from some polyunsaturates extensively recycled into lipid synthesis? *Lipids.* Apr;38(4):477-84, 2003

Fraser DD, Whiting S, Andrew RD, et al, Elevated polyunsaturated fatty acids in blood serum obtained from children on the ketogenic diet. *Neurology.* Mar 25;60(6):1026-9, 2003

Koletzko B, Demmelmair H, Hartl W, et al, The use of stable isotope techniques for nutritional and metabolic research in paediatrics. *Early Hum Dev.* Dec;53 Suppl:S77-97, 1998

McCloy U, Ryan MA, Pencharz PB, et al, A comparison of the metabolism of eighteen-carbon 13C-unsaturated fatty acids in healthy women. *J Lipid Res.* Mar;45(3):474-85, 2004

Brain Plasticity, Memory and Learning

Akbar M, Calderon F, Wen Z, et al, Docosahexaenoic acid: a positive modulator of Akt signaling in neuronal survival. *Proc Natl Acad Sci.* Aug 2;102(31):10858-63, 2005

Bazan NG, Synaptic lipid signaling: significance of polyunsaturated fatty acids and platelet-activating factor. *J Lipid Res.* Dec;44(12):2221-33, 2003

Bazan NG, Lipid signaling in neural plasticity, brain repair, and neuroprotection. *Mol Neurobiol.* Aug;32(1):89-103, 2005

Bazan NG, Neuroprotectin D1 (NPD1): a DHA-derived mediator that protects brain and retina against cell injury-induced oxidative stress. *Brain Pathol.* Apr;15(2):159-66, 2005

Bazan NG, Tu B, Rodriguez de Turco EB, What synaptic lipid signaling tells us about seizure-induced damage and epileptogenesis. *Prog Brain Res.* 135:175-85, 2002

Besana A, Robinson RB, Feinmark SJ, Lipids and two-pore domain K+ channels in excitable cells. *Prostaglandins Other Lipid Mediat.* Sep;77(1-4):103-10, 2005

Cole-Edwards KK, Bazan NG, Lipid signaling in experimental epilepsy. *Neurochem Res.* Jun-Jul;30(6-7):847-53, 2005

Chen C, Bazan NG, Lipid signaling: sleep, synaptic plasticity, and neuroprotection. *Prostaglandins Other Lipid Mediat.* Sep;77(1-4):65-76, 2005

Kuboyama T, Tohda C, Komatsu K, Neuritic regeneration and synaptic reconstruction induced by withanolide A. *Br J Pharmacol.* Apr;144(7):961-71, 2005

Kidd P, Phosphatidylserine: *Nature's Brain Booster for Memory, Mood, and Stress*, St. George: Total Communications, Inc.; 2005

Kidd PM, Neurodegeneration from midochondrial insufficiency: nutrients, stem cells, growth factors, and prospects for brain rebuilding using integrative management. *Altern Med rev.* Dec;10(4):268-93, 2005

Lukiw WJ, Cui JG, Marcheselli VL, et al, A role for docosahexaenoic acid-derived neuroprotectin D1 in neural cell survival and Alzheimer disease. *J Clin Invest.* Oct;115(10):2774-83, 2005

Molteni R, Barnard RJ, Ying Z, et al, A high-fat, refined sugar diet reduces hippocampal brain-derived neurotrophic factor, brain cellal plasticity, and learning. *Neuroscience.* 112(4):803-14, 2002

Popoli M, Gennarelli M, Racagni G, Modulation of synaptic plasticity by stress and antidepressants. *Bipolar Disord.* Jun;4(3):166-82, 2002

Rattiner LM, Davis M, Ressler KJ, Brain-derived neurotrophic factor in amygdala-dependent learning. *Neuroscientist.* Aug;11(4):323-33, 2005

Tyler WJ, Alonso M, Bramham CR, et al, From acquisition to consolidation: on the role of brain-derived neurotrophic factor signaling in hippocampal-dependent learning. *Learn Mem.* Sep-Oct;9(5):224-37, 2002

Wu A, Molteni R, Ying Z, et al, A saturated-fat diet aggravates the outcome of traumatic brain injury on hippocampal plasticity and cognitive function by reducing brain-derived neurotrophic factor. *Neuroscience.* 119(2):365-75, 2003

Wu A, Ying Z, Gomez-Pinilla F, Dietary omega-3 fatty acids normalize BDNF levels, reduce oxidative damage, and counteract learning disability after traumatic brain injury in rats. *J Neurotrauma.* Oct;21(10):1457-67, 2004

Wu A, Ying Z, Gomez-Pinilla F, The interplay between oxidative stress and brain-derived neurotrophic factor modulates the outcome of a saturated fat diet on synaptic plasticity and cognition. *Eur J Neurosci.* Apr;19(7):1699-707, 2004

The "Fat Additction" Theory

Bell SJ, Grochoski GT, Clarke AJ, Health implications of milk containing beta-casein with the A2 genetic variant. *Crit Rev Food Sci Nutr.* 46(1):93-100, 2006

Berger K, Winzell MS, Mei J, et al, Enterostatin and its target mechanisms during regulation of fat intake. *Physiol Behav.* Dec 30;83(4):623-30, 2004

Blass EM, Blom J, beta-Casomorphin causes hypoalgesia in 10-day-old rats: evidence for central mediation. *Pediatr Res.* Feb;39(2):199-203, 1996

Bray GA, Afferent signals regulating food intake. *Proc Nutr Soc.* Aug;59(3):373-84, 2000

Campos H, D'Agostino M, Ordovas JM, Gene-diet interactions and plasma lipoproteins: role of apolipoprotein E and habitual saturated fat intake. *Genet Epidemiol.* Jan;20(1):117-128, 2001

Dubynin VA, Zemskaia NIu, Ivleva IuA, et al, Behavioural effects of beta-casomorphin-7 in its intranasal administration. *Zh Vyssh Nerv Deiat Im I P Pavlova.* May-Jun;54(3):373-81, 2004

Meisel H, FitzGerald RJ, Opioid peptides encrypted in intact milk protein sequences. *Br J Nutr.* Nov;84 Suppl 1:S27-31, 2000

Rizzello CG, Losito I, Gobbetti M, et al, Antibacterial activities of peptides from the water-soluble extracts of Italian cheese varieties. *J Dairy Sci.* Jul;88(7):2348-60, 2005

Sakaguchi M, Koseki M, Wakamatsu M, et al, Effects of systemic administration of beta-casomorphin-5 on learning and memory in mice. *Eur J Pharmacol.* Jan 13;530(1-2):81-7, 2006

Sun Z, Zhang Z, Wang X, et al, Relation of beta-casomorphin to apnea in sudden infant death syndrome. *Peptides.* Jun;24(6):937-43, 2003

Teschemacher H, Koch G, Brantl V, Milk protein-derived opioidreceptor ligands. *Biopolymers.* 43(2):99-117, 1997

CHAPTER FIVE: Smart Proteins: Instant Messengers on the Brain-Wide Web

Amanzadeh J, Gitomer WL, Zerwekh JE, et al, Effect of high protein diet on stone-forming propensity and bone loss in rats. *Kidney Int.* Dec;64(6):2142-9, 2003

Dopamine

Bertolino A, Blasi G, Latorre V, et al, Addictive effects of genetic variation in dopamine regulating genes on working memory cortical activity in human brains. *J Neurosci.* Apr 12;26(15):3918-22, 2006

Bozzi Y, Borrelli E, Dopamine in neurotoxicity and neuroprotection: what do D2 receptors have to do with it? *Trends Neurosci.* Mar;29(3):167-74, 2006

Brunswick DJ, Amsterdam JD, Mozley PD, et al, Greater availability of brain dopamine transporters in major depression shown by [99m Tc]TRODAT-1 SPECT imaging. *Am J Psychiatry.* Oct;160(10):1836-41, 2003

Bustos G, Abarca J, Campusano J, et al, Functional interaction between somatodendritic dopamine release, glutamate receptors and brain-derived neurotrophic factor expression in mesencephalic structures of the brain. *Brain Res Brain Res Rev.* Dec;47(1-3:126-44, 2004

Cocores JA, Dackis CA, Gold MS, Sexual dysfunction secondary to cocaine abuse in two patients. *J Clin Psychiatry.* Jul;47(7):384-5, 1986

Cocores JA, Davies RK, Mueller PS, et al, Cocaine abuse and adult attention deficit disorder. *J Clin Psychiatry.* Sep;48(9):376-7, 1987

Cocores JA, Patel MD, Gold MS, et al, Cocaine abuse, attention deficit disorder, and bipolar disorder. *J Nerv Ment Dis.* Jul;175(7):431-2, 1987

Dewing P, Chiang CW, Sinchak, et al, Direct regulation of adult brain function by the male-specific factor SRY. *Curr Biol.* Feb 21;16(4):415-20, 2006

Eisenberg J, Asnis GM, van Praag HM, et al, Effect of tyrosine on attention deficit disorder with hyperactivity. *J Clin Psychiatry.* May;49(5):193-5, 1988

Erlanson-Albertsson C, How palatable food disrupts appetite regulation. *Basic Clin Pharmacol Toxicol.* Aug;97(2):61-73, 2005

Kienast T, Heinz A, Dopamine and the diseased brain. *CNS Neurol Disord Drug Targets.* Feb;5(1):109-31, 2006

Luo Y, Roth GS, The roles of dopamine oxidative stress and dopamine receptor signaling in aging and age-related neurodegeneration. *Antioxid Redox Signal.* Fall;2(3):449-60, 2000

Mash DC, Pablo J, Ouyang Q, et al, Dopamine transport function is elevated in cocaine users. *J Neurochem.* Apr;81(2):292-300, 2002

Miller NS, Cocores JA, Nicotine dependence: diagnosis, pharmacology and treatment. *J Addict Dis.*11(2):51-65, 1991

Miller NS, Cocores JA, Nicotine dependence: diagnosis, chemistry, and pharmacologic treatments. *Pediatr Rev.* Jul;14(7):275-9, 1993

Salgado-Pineda P, Delaveau P, Blin O, et al, Dopaminergic contribution to the regulation of emotional perception. *Clin Neuropharmacol.* Sep-Oct;28(5):228-37, 2005

Schultz W, Behavioral theories and the neurophysiology of reward. *Annu Rev Psychol.* 57:87-115, 2006

Wang GJ, Volkow ND, Fowler JS, The role of dopamine in motivation for food in humans: implications for obesity. *Expert Opin Ther Targets.* Oct;6(5):601-9,2002

Wang GJ, Volkow ND, Logan J, et al, Brain dopamine and obesity. *Lancet.* Feb3;357(9253):354-7, 2001

Norepineprine

Arnsten AF, Li BM, Neurobiology of executive functions: catecholamine influences on prefrontal cortical functions. *Biol Psychiatry.* Jun 1;57(11):1377-84, 2005

Aston-Jones G, Cohen JD, Adaptive gain and the role of the locus coeruleus-norepinephrine system in optimal performance. *J Comp Neurol.* Dec 5;493(1):99-110, 2005

Bouret S, Sara SJ, Network reset: a simplified overarching theory of locus coeruleus noradrenaline function. *Trends Neurosci.* Nov;28(11):574-82, 2005

Cartford MC, Gould T, Bickford PC. A central role for norepinephrine in the modulation of cerebellar learning tasks. *Behav Cogn Neurosci Rev.* Jun;3(2):131-8, 2004

Nigg JT, Neuropsychologic theory and findings in attention-deficit/hyperactivity disorder: the state of the field and salient challenges for the coming decade. *Biol Psychiatry.* Jun 1;57(11):1424-35, 2005

Tononi G, The neuro-biomolecular basis of alertness in sleep disorders. *Sleep Med.* Jun;6 Suppl 1:S8-12, 2005

Serotonin

Barbas D, DesGroseillers L, Castellucci VF, et al, Multiple serotonergic mechanisms contributing to sensitization in aplysia: evidence of diverse serotonin receptor subtypes. *Learn Mem.* Sep-Oct; 10(5):373-86, 2003

Cocores JA, Miller NS, Pottash AC, et al, Sexual dysfunction in abusers of cocaine and alcohol. *Am J Drug Alcohol Abuse.*14(2):169-73, 1988

Coiro V, Passeri M, Capretti L, et al, Serotonergic control of TSH and PRL secretion in obese men. *Psychoneuroendocrinology.* 15(4):261-8, 1990

Harvey JA., Role of the serotonin 5-HT(2A) receptor in learning. *Learn Mem.* Sep-Oct;10(5):355-62, 2003

Jonas JM, Gold MS, Cocores JA, Phenomenological Link Between Substance Abuse and Eating Disorders. *Society for Neuroscience,* 1986

Martinelli I, Mainini E, Mazzi C, Effect of 5-hydroxytryptophan on the secretion of PRL, GH, TSH and cortisol in obesity. *Minerva Endocrinol.* Jul-Sep;17(3):121-6, 1992

Meneses A, A pharmacological analysis of an associative learning task: 5-HT(1) to 5-HT(7) receptor subtypes function on a pavlovian/instrumental autoshaped memory. *Learn Mem.* Sep-Oct;10(5):363-72, 2003

Mitchell ES, Neumaier JF, 5-HT6 receptors: a novel target for cognitive enhancement. *Pharmacol Ther.* Dec;108(3):320-33, 2005

Glutamate

Butterfield DA, Pocernich CB. The glutamatergic system and Alzheimer's disease: therapeutic implications. *CNS Drugs.* 17(9):641-52, 2003

Daoudal G, Debanne D, Long-term plasticity of intrinsic excitability: learning rules and mechanisms. *Learn Mem.* Nov-Dec;10(6):456-65, 2003

Gould TJ, Lewis MC, Coantagonism of glutamate receptors and nicotinic acetylcholinergic receptors disrupts fear conditioning and latent inhibition of fear conditioning. *Learn Mem.* Jul-Aug;12(4):389-98, 2005

Helms G, Ciumas C, Kyaga S, et al, Increased thalamus levels of glutamate and glutamine (Glx) in patients with idiopathic generalised epilepsy. *J Neurol Neurosurg Psychiatry.* Apr;77(4):489-94, 2006

Holscher C, Schmid S, Pilz PK, Lack of the metabotropic glutamate receptor subtype 7 selectively modulates Theta rhythm and working memory. *Learn Mem.* Sep-Oct;12(5):450-5, 2005

Sullivan JM, Cellular and molecular mechanisms underlying learning and memory impairments produced by cannabinoids. *Learn Mem.* May-Jun;7(3):132-9, 2000

Zacco A, Togo J, Spence K, et al, 3-hydroxy-3-methylglutaryl coenzyme A reductase inhibitors protect cortical brain cells from excitotoxicity. *J Neurosci.* Dec 3;23(35):11104-11, 2003

Glycine

Barch DM, Pharmacological manipulation of human working memory. *Psychopharmacology (Berl).* Jun;174(1):126-35, 2004

Cervo L, Cocco A, Carnovali F, Effects on cocaine and food self-administration of (+)-HA-966, a partial agonist at the glycine/NMDA modulatory site, in rats. *Psychopharmacology (Berl).* Apr;173(1-2):124-31, 2004

File SE, Fluck E, Fernandes C, Beneficial effects of glycine (bioglycin) on memory and attention in young and middle-aged adults. *J Clin Psychopharmacol.* Dec;19(6):506-12, 1999

Saul'skaya NB, Solov'eva NA, Tetrodotoxin-dependent glycine release in the rat nucleus accumbens during correction of feeding behavior. *Neurosci Behav Physiol.* Oct;35(8):815-9, 2005

GABA

Backstrom T, Andersson A, Andree L, et al, Pathogenesis in menstrual cycle-linked CNS disorders. *Ann N Y Acad Sci.* Dec;1007:42-53, 2003

Birzniece V, Backstrom T, Johansson IM, et al, Neuroactive steroid effects on cognitive functions with a focus on the serotonin and GABA systems. *Brain Res Brain Res Rev.* Dec 17, 2005

Dougherty JA, Rhoney DH, Gabapentin: a unique anti-epileptic agent. *Neurol Res.* Dec;23(8):821-9, 2001

Petty F, Davis LL, Kabel D, et al, Serotonin dysfunction disorders: a behavioral neurochemistry perspective. *J Clin Psychiatry.* 57 Suppl 8:11-6, 1996

Zarrindast MR, Noorbakhshnia M, Motamedi F, et al, Effect of the GABAergic system on memory formation and state-dependent learning induced by morphine in rats. *Pharmacology.* 76(2):93-100, 2006

Acetylcholine

Ballard CG, Greig NH, Guillozet-Bongaarts AL, et al, Cholinesterases: roles in the brain during health and disease. *Curr Alzheimer Res.* Jul;2(3):307-18, 2005

Beane M, Marrocco RT, Norepinephrine and acetylcholine mediation of the components of reflexive attention: implications for attention deficit disorders. *Prog Neurobiol.* Oct;74(3):167-81, 2004

Buccafusco JJ, Letchworth SR, Bencherif M, et al, Long-lasting cognitive improvement with nicotinic receptor agonists: mechanisms of pharmacokinetic-pharmacodynamic discordance. *Trends Pharmacol Sci.* Jul;26(7):352-60, 2005

Gold PE, Coordination of multiple memory systems. Neurobiol *Learn Mem.* Nov;82(3):230-42, 2004

Narahashi T, Moriguchi S, Zhao X, et al, Mechanisms of action of cognitive enhancers on neuroreceptors. *Biol Pharm Bull.* Nov;27(11):1701-6, 2004

Rosecrans JA, *The Biobehavioral Effects of Nicotine, In The Clinical Management of Nicotine Dependence,* JA Cocores (Editor), 53-65, 1991

Souder E, Neuropathology in Alzheimer's disease: target of pharmacotherapy. *J Am Acad Nurse Pract.* Mar;Suppl:3-5, 2005

Adenosine

Lorist MM, Tops M, Caffeine, fatigue, and cognition. *Brain Cogn.* Oct;53(1):82-94, 2003

Ribeiro JA, Sebastiao AM, Mendonca A, Participation of adenosine receptors in neuroprotection. *Drug News Perspect.* Mar;16(2) 80-6, 2003

Rose GM, Hopper A, De Vivo M, et al, Phosphodiesterase inhibitors for cognitive enhancement. *Curr Pharm Des.* 11(26):3329-34, 2005

Endorphins

Aktas G, Ogce F, Dance as a therapy for cancer prevention. *Asian Pac J Cancer Prev.* Jul-Sep; 6(3):408-11, 2005

Esch T, Stefano GB, The neurobiology of pleasure, reward processes, addiction and their health implications. *Neuro Endocrinol Lett.* Aug;25(4):235-51, 2004

Fobes JL, The cognitive psychobiology of performance regulation. *J Sports Med Phys Fitness.* Jun;29(2):202-8, 1989

Guieu R, Devaux C, Albanese J, et al, Beta-endorphin in multiple trauma victims. *Can J Neurol Sci.* May;22(2):160-3, 1995

Hebb AL, Poulin JF, Roach SP, et al, Cholecystokinin and endogenous opioid peptides: interactive influence on pain, cognition, and emotion. *Prog Neuropsychopharmacol Biol Psychiatry.* Dec;29(8):1225-38, 2005

Kelley AE, Baldo BA, Pratt WE, et al, Corticostriatal-hypothalamic circuitry and food motivation: integration of energy, action and reward. *Physiol Behav.* Dec 15;86(5):773-95, 2005

CCK

Benedetti F, Amanzio M, The neurobiology of placebo analgesia: from endogenous opioids to cholecystokinin. *Prog Neurobiol.* Jun;52(2):109-25, 1997

Bradwejn J, Koszycki D, Cholecystokinin and panic disorder: past and future clinical research strategies. *Scand J Clin Lab Invest Suppl.* 234:19-27, 2001

Dauge V, Lena I, CCK in anxiety and cognitive processes. *Neurosci Biobehav Rev.* Oct;22(6): 815-25, 1998

Donini LM, Savina C, Cannella C, Eating habits and appetite control in the elderly: the anorexia of aging. *Int Psychogeriatr.* Mar;15(1):73-87, 2003

Gulpinar MA, Yegen BC, The physiology of learning and memory: role of peptides and stress. *Curr Protein Pept Sci.* Dec;5(6):457-73, 2004

Hadjiivanova C, Belcheva S, Belcheva I, Cholecystokinin and learning and memory processes. Acta *Physiol Pharmacol Bulg.* 27(2-3):83-8, 2003

Soy Protein

Buzalaf MA, Damante CA, Trevizani LM, et al, Risk of fluorosis associated with infant formulas prepared with bottled water. *J Dent Child (Chic).* May-Aug;71(2):110-3, 2004

Chen J, Shan KR, Long YG, et al, Selective decreases of nicotinic acetylcholine receptors in PC12 cells exposed to fluoride. *Toxicology.* Feb 1;183(1-3):235-42, 2003

Cockell KA, Bonacci G, Belonje B, Manganese content of soy or rice beverages is high in comparison to infant formulas. *J Am Coll Nutr.* Apr;23(2):124-30, 2004

Collipp PJ, Chen SY, Maitinsky S, Manganese in infant formulas and learning disability. *Ann Nutr Metab.* 27(6):488-94, 1983

Fernandez-Lorenzo JR, Cocho JA, Rey-Goldar ML, et al, Aluminum contents of human milk, cow's milk, and infant formulas. *J Pediatr Gastroenterol Nutr.* Mar;28(3):270-5, 1999

Foucard T, Malmheden Yman I, A study on severe food reactions in Sweden-is soy protein an underestimated cause of food anaphylaxis? *Allergy.* Mar;54(3):261-5, 1999

Golub MS, Hogrefe CE, Germann SL, et al, Neurobehavioral evaluation of rhesus monkey infants fed cow's milk formula, soy formula, or soy formula with added manganese. *Neurotoxicol Teratol.* Jul-Aug;27(4):615-27, 2005

Grant G, Anti-nutritional effects of soyabean: a review. *Prog Food Nutr Sci.* 13(3-4):317-48, 1989

Grant G, Dorward PM, Pusztai A, Pancreatic enlargement is evident in rats fed diets containing raw soybeans (Glycine max) or cowpeas (Vigna unguiculata) for 800 days but not in those fed diets based on kidney beans (Phaseolus vulgaris) or lupinseed (Lupinus angustifolius). *J Nutr.* Dec;123(12):2207-15, 1993

Greger JL, Dietary and other sources of aluminium intake. *Ciba Found Symp.* 169:26-35; discussion 35-49, 1992

Karagas MR, Baron JA, Barrett JA, et al, Patterns of fracture among the United States elderly: geographic and fluoride effects. *Ann Epidemiol.* May;6(3):209-16, 1996

Koo WW, Kaplan LA, Krug-Wispe SK, Aluminum contamination of infant formulas. *JPEN J Parenter Enteral Nutr.* Mar-Apr;12(2):170-3, 1988

Inomata N, Osuna H, Yanagimachi M, et al, Late-onset anaphylaxis to fermented soybeans: the first confirmation of food-induced, late-onset anaphylaxis by provocation test. *Ann Allergy Asthma Immunol.* Mar;94(3):402-6, 2005

Levison DA, Morgan RG, Brimacombe JS, et al, Carcinogenic effects of Di(2-hydroxypropyl)nitrosamine (DHPN) in male Wistar rats: promotion of pancreatic cancer by a raw soya flour diet. *Scand J Gastroenterol.* 14(2):217-24, 1979

Li Z, Li D, Qiao S, et al, Anti-nutritional effects of a moderate dose of soybean agglutinin in the rat. *Arch Tierernahr.* Aug;57(4):267-77, 2003

Massey LK, Palmer RG, Horner HT, Oxalate content of soybean seeds (Glycine max: Leguminosae), soyfoods, and other edible legumes. *J Agric Food Chem.* Sep;49(9):4262-6, 2001

McGuinness EE, Wormsley KG, Effects of feeding partial and intermittent raw soya flour diets on the rat pancreas. *Cancer Lett.* Jul;32(1):73-81, 1986

Mills EN, Breiteneder H, Food allergy and its relevance to industrial food proteins. *Biotechnol Adv.* Sep;23(6):409-14, 2005

Nishikawa A, Ikeda T, Son HY, et al, Pronounced synergistic promotion of N-bis(2-hydroxypropyl)nitrosamine-initiated thyroid tumorigenesis in rats treated with excess soybean and iodine-deficient diets. *Toxicol Sci.* Aug;86(2):258-63, 2005

Palacios MF, Easter RA, Soltwedel KT, et al, Effect of soybean variety and processing on growth performance of young chicks and pigs. *J Anim Sci.* Apr;82(4):1108-14, 2004

Pusztai A, Grant G, Bardocz S, et al, Novel dietary strategy for overcoming the antinutritional effects of soyabean whey of high agglutinin content. *Br J Nutr.* Jun;77(6):933-45, 1997

Simons E, Weiss CC, Furlong TJ, et al, Impact of ingredient labeling practices on food allergic consumers. *Ann Allergy Asthma Immunol.* Nov;95(5):426-8, 2005

van der Voet GB, Schijns O, de Wolff FA, Fluoride enhances the effect of aluminium chloride on interconnections between aggregates of hippocampal brain cells. *Arch Physiol Biochem.* Feb;107(1): 15-21, 1999

Whey

Boehm G, Cervantes H, Georgi G, et al, Effect of increasing dietary threonine intakes on amino acid metabolism of the central nervous system and peripheral tissues in growing rats. *Pediatr Res.* Dec;44(6):900-6, 1998

Boza JJ, Moennoz D, Jarret AR, et al, Neither glutamine nor arginine supplementation of diets increase glutamine body stores in healthy growing rats. *Clin Nutr.* Oct;19(5):319-25, 2000

Desrosiers T, Savoie L, Extent of damage to amino acid availability of whey protein heated with sugar. *J Dairy Res.* Nov;58(4):431-41, 1991

Fanaro S, Vigi V, Protein quality and quantity in infant formulas. A critical look. *Minerva Pediatr.* Jun;54(3):203-9, 2002

Gleeson M, Interrelationship between physical activity and branched-chain amino acids. *J Nutr.* Jun;135(6 Suppl):1591S-5S, 2005

Lambert CP, Frank LL, Evans WJ, Macronutrient considerations for the sport of bodybuilding. *Sports Med.* 34(5):317-27, 2004

Lonnerdal B, Effects of milk and milk components on calcium, magnesium, and trace element absorption during infancy. *Physiol Rev.* Jul;77(3):643-69, 1997

Marshall K, Therapeutic applications of whey protein. *Altern Med Rev.* Jun;9(2):136-56, 2004

Mucchetti G, Locci F, Gatti M, et al, Pyroglutamic acid in cheese: presence, origin, and correlation with ripening time of Grana Padano cheese. *J Dairy Sci.* Apr;83(4):659-65, 2000

Penttila IA, Zhang MF, Bates E, et al, Immune modulation in suckling rat pups by a growth factor extract derived from milk whey. *J Dairy Res.* Nov;68(4):587-99, 2001

Phillips SM, Hartman JW, Wilkinson SB, Dietary protein to support anabolism with resistance exercise in young men. *J Am Coll Nutr.* Apr;24(2):134S-139S, 2005

Rassin DK, Gaull GE, Heinonen K, et al, Milk protein quantity and quality in low-birth-weight infants: II. Effects on selected aliphatic amino acids in plasma and urine. *Pediatrics.* Mar;59(3):407-22, 1977

Rutherfurd KJ, Gill HS, Peptides affecting coagulation. *Br J Nutr.* Nov;84 Suppl 1:S99-102, 2000

Cheese

Boeing H, Epidemiological research in stomach cancer: progress over the last ten years. *J Cancer Res Clin Oncol.* 117(2):133-43, 1991

Iishi H, Tatsuta M, Baba M, et al, Low-protein diet promotes sodium chloride-enhanced gastric carcinogenesis induced by N-methyl-N'-nitro-N-nitrosoguanidine in Wistar rats. *Cancer Lett.* Jul 1;141(1-2):117-22, 1999

Lee JK, Park BJ, Yoo KY, et al, Dietary factors and stomach cancer: a case-control study in Korea. *Int J Epidemiol.* Feb;24(1):33-41, 1995

Sugimura T, Wakabayashi K, Gastric carcinogenesis: diet as a causative factor. *Med Oncol Tumor Pharmacother.* 7(2-3):87-92, 1990

Tatematsu M, Takahashi M, Fukushima S, et al, Effects in rats of sodium chloride on experimental gastric cancers induced by N-methyl-N-nitro-N-nitrosoguanidine or 4-nitroquinoline-1-oxide. *J Natl Cancer Inst.* Jul;55(1):101-6, 1975

Mercury in Fish

Castoldi AF, Coccini T, Neurotoxic and molecular effects of methylmercury in humans. *Rev Environ Health.* Jan-Mar;18(1):19-31, 2003

Chan HM, Egeland GM, Fish consumption, mercury exposure, and heart diseases. *Nutr Rev.* Feb;62(2):68-72, 2004

Hansen JC, Gilman AP, Exposure of Arctic populations to methylmercury from consumption of marine food: an updated risk-benefit assessment. *Int J Circumpolar Health.* Apr;64(2):121-36, 2005

Kazantzis G, Mercury exposure and early effects: an overview. *Med Lav.* May-Jun;93(3):139-47, 2002

Kidd PM, Neurodegeneration from mitochondrial insufficiency: nutrients, stem cells, growth factors, and prospects for brain rebuilding using integrative management. *Altern Med Rev.* Dec;10(4):268-93, 2005

Mahaffey KR, Fish and shellfish as dietary sources of methylmercury and the omega-3 fatty acids, eicosahexaenoic acid and docosahexaenoic acid: risks and benefits. *Environ Res.* Jul;95(3):414-28, 2004

Mahaffey KR, Methylmercury: a new look at the risks. *Public Health Rep.* Sep-Oct;114(5):396-9, 402-13, 1999

Risher JF, Murray HE, Prince GR, Organic mercury compounds: human exposure and its relevance to public health. *Toxicol Ind Health.* Apr;18(3):109-60, 2002

Sanfeliu C, Sebastia J, Cristofol R, et al, Neurotoxicity of organomercurial compounds. *Neurotox Res.* 5(4):283-305, 2003

Shanker G, Syversen T, Aschner JL, et al, Modulatory effect of glutathione status and antioxidants on methylmercury-induced free radical formation in primary cultures of cerebral astrocytes. *Brain Res Mol Brain Res.* Jun 13;137(1-2):11-22, 2005

Smith KM, Sahyoun NR, Fish consumption: recommendations versus advisories, can they be reconciled? *Nutr Rev.* Feb;63(2):39-46, 2005

Valko M, Morris H, Cronin MT, Metals, toxicity and oxidative stress. *Curr Med Chem.* 12(10):1161-208, 2005

Watanabe C, Selinium deficiency and brain functions: the significance for methylmercury toxicity. *Nippon Eiseigaku Zasshi,* Jan;55(4):581-9, 2001

Dioxins/PCBs

Carney SA, Prasch AL, Heideman W, et al, Understanding dioxin developmental toxicity using the zebrafish model. *Birth Defects Res A Clin Mol Teratol.* Jan;76(1):7-18, 2006

Hays SM, Aylward LL, Dioxin risks in perspective: past, present, and future. *Regul Toxicol Pharmacol.* Apr;37(2):202-17, 2003

Hites RA, Foran JA, Carpenter DO, Global assessment of organic contaminants in farmed salmon. *Science.* Jan 9;303(5655):226-9, 2004

Needham LL, Barr DB, Caudill SP, et al, Concentrations of environmental chemicals associated with neurodevelopmental effects in U.S. population. *Neurotoxicology.* Aug;26(4):531-45, 2005

Popp JA, Crouch E, McConnell EE, A Weight-of-evidence analysis of the cancer dose-response characteristics of 2,3,7,8-tetrachlorodibenzodioxin (TCDD). *Toxicol Sci.* Feb;89(2):361-9, 2006

Schwarz M, Appel KE, Carcinogenic risks of dioxin: mechanistic considerations. *Regul Toxicol Pharmacol.* Oct;43(1):19-34, 2005

Sher ES, Xu XM, Adams PM, The effects of thyroid hormone level and action in developing brain: are these targets for the actions of polychlorinated biphenyls and dioxins? *Toxicol Ind Health.* Jan-Apr;14(1-2):121-58, 1998

Vreugdenhil HJ, Lanting CI, Mulder PG, et al, Effects of prenatal PCB and dioxin background exposure on cognitive and motor abilities in Dutch children at school age. *J Pediatr.* Jan;140(1):48-56, 2002

The Protein Addiction Theory

Drewnowski A, Krahn DD, Demitrack MA, et al, Taste responses and preferences for sweet high-fat foods: evidence for opioid involvement. *Physiol Behav.* Feb;51(2):371-9, 1992

Gin H, Rigalleau V, Aparicio M, Lipids, protein intake, and diabetic nephropathy. *Diabetes Metab.* Jul;26 Suppl 4:45-53, 2000

Holt SH, Miller JC, Petocz P, An insulin index of foods: the insulin demand generated by 1000-kJ portions of common foods. *Am J Clin Nutr.* Nov;66(5):1264-76, 1997

James JS, Marijuana and chocolate. *AIDS Treat News.* Oct 18;(No 257):3-4, 1996

Kalra SP, Kalra PS, Overlapping and interactive pathways regulating appetite and craving. *J Addict Dis.* 23(3):5-21, 2004

Tabuchi E, Ono T, Nishijo, et al, Amino acid and NaCl appetite, and LHA neuron responses of lysine-deficient rat. *Physiol Behav.* May;49(5):951-64, 1991

Veldhuis WB, van der Stelt M, Wadman MW, et al, Neuroprotection by the endogenous cannabinoid anandamide and arvanil against in vivo excitotoxicity in the rat: role of vanilloid receptors and lipoxygenases. *J Neurosci.* May 15;23(10):4127-33, 2003

Wang GJ, Volkow ND, Logan J, et al, Brain dopamine and obesity. *Lancet,* Feb 3;357(9253):354-7, 2001

Wang GJ, Volkow ND, Thanos PK, et al, Similarity between obesity and drug addicition as assessed by neurofunctional imaging. *J Addict Dis.* 23(3):39-53, 2004

Yanovski S, Sugar and fat: cravings and aversions. *J Nutr.* Mar;133(3):835S-837S, 2003

Yeomans MR, Gray RW, Selective effects of naltrexone on food pleasantness and intake. *Physiol Behav.* Aug;60(2):439-46, 1996

Yeomans MR, Wright P, Macleod HA, et al, Effects of nalmefene on feeding in humans. Dissociation of hunger and palatability. *Psychopharmacology* 100(3):426-32, 1990

CHAPTER SIX: Slowly Absorbed Glucose: High-Speed Access to Well-Being

Glucose is a Star

Aberg ND, Brywe KG, Isgaard J, Aspects of growth hormone and insulin-like growth factor-I related to neuroprotection, regeneration, and functional plasticity in the adult brain. *ScientificWorldJournal.* Jan 18;6:53-80, 2006

Dye L, Lluch A, Blundell JE, Macronutrients and mental performance. *Nutrition.* Oct;16(10):1021-34, 2000

Greenwood CE, Dietary carbohydrate, glucose regulation, and cognitive performance in elderly persons. *Nutr Rev.* May;61(5 Pt 2):S68-74, 2003

Gold PE, Role of glucose in regulating the brain and cognition. *Am J Clin Nutr.* Apr;61(4 Suppl):987S-995S, 1995

Korol DL, Gold PE, Glucose, memory, and aging. *Am J Clin Nutr.* Apr;67(4):764S-771S, 1998

Manning CA, Stone WS, Korol DL, et al, Glucose enhancement of 24-h memory retrieval in healthy elderly humans. *Behav Brain Res.* Jun;93(1-2):71-6, 1998

Marvel CL, Paradiso S, Cognitive and neurological impairment in mood disorders. *Psychiatr Clin North Am.* Mar;27(1):19-36, vii-viii, 2004

Messier C, Glucose improvement of memory: a review. *Eur J Pharmacol.* Apr 19;490(1-3):33-57, 2004

Riby LM, McMurtrie H, Smallwood J, et al, The facilitative effects of glucose ingestion on memory retrieval in younger and older adults: is task difficulty or task domain critical? *Br J Nutr.* Feb;95(2): 414-20, 2006

Ryan CM, Freed MI, Rood JA, et al, Improving metabolic control leads to better working memory in adults with type 2 diabetes. *Diabetes Care.* Feb;29(2):345-51, 2006

Sonntag WE, Ramsey M, Carter CS, Growth hormone and insulin-like growth factor-1 (IGF-1) and their influence on cognitive aging. *Ageing Res Rev.* May;4(2):195-212, 2005

Valiante AG, Barr RG, Zelazo PR, et al, A typical feeding enhances memory for spoken words in healthy 2- to 3-day-old newborns. *Pediatrics.* Mar;117(3):e476-86, 2006

Vogt BA, Laureys S, Posterior cingulate, precuneal and retrosplenial cortices: cytology and components of the neural network correlates of consciousness. *Prog Brain Res.* 150:205-17, 2005

Wang GJ, Volkow ND, Thanos PK, et al, Similarity between obesity and drug addiction as assessed by neurofunctioning imaging: a concept review. *J Addict Dis.* 23(3):39-53, 2004

White JW, Wolraich M, Effect of sugar on behavior and mental performance. *Am J Clin Nutr.* Jul;62(1 Suppl):242S-247S, 1995

Wolraich ML, Wilson DB, White JW, The effect of sugar on behavior or cognition in children. A meta-analysis. *JAMA.* Nov 22-29;274(20):1617-21, 1995

Rapidly-Absorbed Glucose and Power Surges

Awad N, Gagnon M, Messier C, The relationship between impaired glucose tolerance, type 2 diabetes, and cognitive function. *J Clin Exp Neuropsychol.* Nov;26(8):1044-80, 2004

Burcelin R, The incretins: a link between nutrients and well-being. *Br J Nutr.* Apr;93 Suppl 1:S147-56, 2005

Cox D, Gonder-Frederick L, McCall A, et al, The effects of glucose fluctuation on cognitive function and QOL: the functional costs of hypoglycaemia and hyperglycaemia among adults with type 1 or type 2 diabetes. *Int J Clin Pract Suppl.* Jul;(129):20-6, 2002

Cox DJ, Kovatchev BP, Gonder-Frederick LA, et al, Relationships between hyperglycemia and cognitive performance among adults with type 1 and type 2 diabetes. *Diabetes Care.* Jan;28(1):71-7, 2005

Gispen WH, Biessels GJ, Cognition and synaptic plasticity in diabetes mellitus. *Trends Neurosci.* Nov;23(11):542-9, 2000

Launer LJ, Diabetes and brain aging: epidemiologic evidence. *Curr Diab Rep.* Feb;5(1):59-63, 2005

Li ZG, Sima AA, C-peptide and central nervous system complications in diabetes. *Exp Diabesity Res.* Jan-Mar;5(1):79-90, 2004

Polonsky WH, Davis CL, Jacobson AM, et al, Hyperglycaemia, hypoglycaemia, and blood glucose control in diabetes: symptom perceptions and treatment strategies. *Diabet Med.* Mar;9(2):120-5, 1992

Sima AA, Kamiya H, Li ZG, Insulin, C-peptide, hyperglycemia, and central nervous system complications in diabetes. *Eur J Pharmacol.* Apr 19;490(1-3):187-97, 2004

Sommerfield AJ, Deary IJ, Frier BM, Acute hyperglycemia alters mood state and impairs cognitive performance in people with type 2 diabetes. *Diabetes Care.* Oct;27(10):233540, 2004

Brown-Outs

Bober E, Buyukgebiz A, Hypoglycemia and its effects on the brain in children with type 1 diabetes mellitus. *Pediatr Endocrinol Rev.* Mar;2(3):378-82, 2005

Bojanowska E, Physiology and pathophysiology of glucagon-like peptide-1 (GLP-1): the role of GLP-1 in the pathogenesis of diabetes mellitus, obesity, and stress. *Med Sci Monit.* Aug;11(8):RA271-8, 2005

Cheyne EH, Sherwin RS, Lunt MJ, et al, Influence of alcohol on cognitive performance during mild hypoglycaemia; implications for Type 1 diabetes. *Diabet Med.* Mar;21(3):230-7, 2004

Cox D, Clarke W, Gonder-Frederick L, et al, Driving mishaps and hypoglycaemia: risk and prevention. *Int J Clin Pract Suppl.* Sep;(123):38-42, 2001

Davis S, Alonso MD, Hypoglycemia as a barrier to glycemic control. *J Diabetes Complications.* Jan-Feb;18(1):60-8, 2004 de la Monte SM, Wands JR, Review of insulin and insulin-like growth factor expression, signaling, and malfunction in the central nervous system: relevance to Alzheimer's disease. *J Alzheimers Dis.* Feb;7(1):45-61, 2005

Desrocher M, Rovet J, Neurocognitive correlates of type 1 diabetes mellitus in childhood. *Neuropsychol Dev Cogn C Child Neuropsychol.* Mar;10(1):36-52, 2004

Fanelli CG, Pampanelli S, Porcellati F, et al, Rate of fall of blood glucose and physiological responses of counterregulatory hormones, clinical symptoms and cognitive function to hypoglycaemia in Type I diabetes mellitus in the postprandial state. *Diabetologia.* Jan;46(1):53-64, 2003

Frier BM, Hypoglycaemia and cognitive function in diabetes. *Int J Clin Pract Suppl.* Sep;(123):30-7, 2001

Graveling AJ, Warren RE, Frier BM, et al, Hypoglycaemia and driving in people with insulin-treated diabetes: adherence to recommendations for avoidance. *Diabet Med.* Sep;21(9):1014-9, 2004

Kouta Y, Sakurai T, Yokono K, Cognitive dysfunction and dementia associated with elderly diabetes. *Nippon Rinsho.* Jan;64(1):119-23, 2006

Lustman PJ, Clouse RE, Depression in diabetic patients: the relationship between mood and glycemic control. *J Diabetes Complications.* Mar-Apr;19(2):113-22, 2005

McNay EC, The impact of recurrent hypoglycemia on cognitive function in aging. *Neurobiol Aging.* Dec;26 Suppl 1:76-9, 2005

Messier C, Teutenberg K, The role of insulin, insulin growth factor, and insulin-degrading enzyme in brain aging and Alzheimer's disease. *Neural Plast.* 12(4):311-28, 2005

Mosconi L, Brain glucose metabolism in the early and specific diagnosis of Alzheimer's disease. FDG-PET studies in MCI and AD. *Eur J Nucl Med Mol Imaging.* Apr;32(4):486-510, 2005

Plum L, Schubert M, Bruning JC, The role of insulin receptor signaling in the brain. Trends *Endocrinol Metab.* Mar;16(2):59-65, 2005

Rapoport SI, Hatanpaa K, Brady DR, et al, Brain energy metabolism, cognitive function and down-regulated oxidative phosphorylation in Alzheimer disease. *Neurodegeneration.* Dec;5(4):473-6, 1996

Silverman DH, Alavi A, PET imaging in the assessment of normal and impaired cognitive function. *Radiol Clin North Am.* Jan;43(1):67-77, 2005

Smitz S, The care of the older person with diabetes mellitus. *Rev Med Liege.* May-Jun;60(5-6):433-8, 2005

Strachan MW, Ewing FM, Frier BM, et al, Effects of acute hypoglycaemia on auditory information processing in adults with Type I diabetes. *Diabetologia.* Jan;46(1):97-105, 2003

Warren RE, Frier BM, Hypoglycaemia and cognitive function. *Diabetes Obes Metab.* Sep;7(5): 493-503, 2005

The "Rapidly- and Moderately-Absorbed Glucose Addiction" Theory

Amit Z, Galina ZH, Stress induced analgesia plays an adaptive role in the organization of behavioral responding. *Brain Res Bull.* Dec;21(6):955-8, 1988

Kracke GR, Uthoff KA, Tobias JD, et al, Sugar solution analgesia: the effects of glucose on expressed mu opioid receptors. *Anesth Analg.* Jul;101(1):64-8, 2005

Leibowitz SF, Alexander JT, Hypothalamic serotonin in control of eating behavior, meal size, and body weight. *Biol Psychiatry.* Nov 1;44(9):851-64, 1998

Takahashi M, Fukunaga H, Kaneto H, et al, Behavioral and pharmacological studies on gluten exorphin A5, a newly isolated bioactive food protein fragment, in mice. *Jpn J Pharmacol.* Nov;84(3):259-65, 2000

Wurtman RJ, Wurtman JJ, Brain serotonin, carbohydrate-craving, obesity and depression. *Obes Res.* Nov;3 Suppl 4:477S-480S, 1995

Yoshikawa M, Takahashi M, Yang S, Delta opioid peptides derived from plant proteins. *Curr Pharm Des.* 9(16):1325-30, 2003

Slowly-Absorbed Glucose Workshop

Ball SD, Keller KR, Moyer-Mileur LJ, et al, Prolongation of satiety after low versus moderately high glycemic index meals in obese adolescents. *Pediatrics.* Mar;111(3):488-94, 2003

Belderson P, Harvey I, Kimbell R, et al, Does breakfast-club attendance affect schoolchildren's nutrient intake? A study of dietary intake at three schools. *Br J Nutr.* Dec;90(6):1003-6, 2003

Bell SJ, Sears B, Low-glycemic-load diets: impact on obesity and chronic diseases. *Crit Rev Food Sci Nutr.* 43(4):357-77, 2003

Benton D, Nabb S, Breakfasts that release glucose at different speeds interact with previous alcohol intake to influence cognition and mood before and after lunch. *Behav Neurosci.* Oct;118(5):936-43, 2004

Benton D, Ruffin MP, Lassel T, et al, The delivery rate of dietary carbohydrates affects cognitive performance in both rats and humans. *Psychopharmacology* Feb;166(1):86-90, 2003

Bjorck I, Elmstahl HL, The glycaemic index: importance of dietary fibre and other food properties. *Proc Nutr Soc.* Feb;62(1):201-6, 2003

Brand-Miller JC, Glycemic load and chronic disease. *Nutr Rev.* May;61(5 Pt 2):S49-55, 2003

Briggs M, Safaii S, Beall DL, Position of the American Dietetic Association, Society for Nutrition Education, and American School Food Service Association-Nutrition services: an essential component of comprehensive school health programs. *J Am Diet Assoc.* Apr;103(4):505-14, 2003

Brynes AE, Mark Edwards C, Ghatei MA, et al, A randomised four-intervention crossover study investigating the effect of carbohydrates on daytime profiles of insulin, glucose, non-esterified fatty acids and triacylglycerols in middle-aged men. *Br J Nutr.* Feb;89(2):207-18, 2003

Buyken AE, Dettmann W, Kersting M, et al, Glycaemic index and glycaemic load in the diet of healthy schoolchildren: trends from 1990 to 2002, contribution of different carbohydrate sources and relationships to dietary quality. *Br J Nutr.* Nov;94(5):796-803, 2005

Cueto S, Breakfast and performance. *Public Health Nutr.* Dec;4(6A):1429-31, 2001

Dickinson S, Brand-Miller J, Glycemic index, postprandial glycemia and cardiovascular disease. *Curr Opin Lipidol.* Feb;16(1):69-75, 2005

Flint A, Moller BK, Raben A, et al, The use of glycaemic index tables to predict glycaemic index of composite breakfast meals. *Br J Nutr.* Jun;91(6):979-89, 2004

Foster-Powell K, Holt SH, Brand-Miller JC, International table of glycemic index and glycemic load values. *Am J Clin Nutr.* Jul;76(1):5-56, 2002

Grantham-McGregor S, Can the provision of breakfast benefit school performance? *Food Nutr Bull.* Jun;26(2 Suppl 2):S144-58, 2005

Gross SM, Cinelli B, Coordinated school health program and dietetics professionals: partners in promoting healthful eating. *J Am Diet Assoc.* May;104(5):793-8, 2004

Jimenez-Cruz A, Bacardi-Gascon M, Turnbull WH, et al, A flexible, low-glycemic index mexican-style diet in overweight and obese subjects with type 2 diabetes improves metabolic parameters during a 6-week treatment period. *Diabetes Care.* Jul;26(7):1967-70, 2003

Kelly S, Frost G, Whittaker V, et al, Low glycaemic index diets for coronary heart disease. *Cochrane Database Syst Rev.* Oct 18;(4):CD004467, 2004

Kimura S, Glycemic carbohydrate and health: background and synopsis of the symposium. *Nutr Rev.* May;61(5 Pt 2):S1-4, 2003

Kleinman RE, Hall S, Green H, et al, Diet, breakfast, and academic performance in children. *Ann Nutr Metab.* 46 Suppl 1:24-30, 2002

Korol DL, Enhancing cognitive function across the life span. *Ann N Y Acad Sci.* Apr;959:167-79, 2002

Livesey G, Low-glycaemic diets and health: implications for obesity. *Proc Nutr Soc.* Feb;64(1):105-13, 2005

Mahoney CR, Taylor HA, Kanarek RB, et al, Effect of breakfast composition on cognitive processes in elementary school children. *Physiol Behav.* Aug 7;85(5):635-45, 2005

Monro JA, Glycaemic glucose equivalent: combining carbohydrate content, quantity and glycaemic index of foods for precision in glycaemia management. *Asia Pac J Clin Nutr.* 11(3):217-25, 2002

Moyad MA, Fad diets and obesity-Part IV: Low-carbohydrate vs. low-fat diets. *Urol Nurs.* Feb; 25(1):67-70, 2005

Murphy JM, Pagano ME, Nachmani J, et al, The relationship of school breakfast to psychosocial and academic functioning: cross-sectional and longitudinal observations in an inner-city school sample. *Arch Pediatr Adolesc Med.* Sep;152(9):899-907, 1998

Nabb S, Benton D, The influence on cognition of the interaction between the macro-nutrient content of breakfast and glucose tolerance. *Physiol Behav.* Jan 30;87(1):16-23, 2006

Opperman AM, Venter CS, Oosthuizen W, et al, Meta-analysis of the health effects of using the glycaemic index in meal-planning. *Br J Nutr.* Sep;92(3):367-81, 2004

Pawlak DB, Kushner JA, Ludwig DS, Effects of dietary glycaemic index on adiposity, glucose homoeostasis, and plasma lipids in animals. *Lancet.* Aug 28-Sep 3;364(9436):778-85, 2004

Pilant VB, Position of the American Dietetic Association: local support for nutrition integrity in schools. *J Am Diet Assoc.* Jan;106(1):122-33, 2006

Pollitt E, Cueto S, Jacoby ER, Fasting and cognition in well- and undernourished schoolchildren: a review of three experimental studies. *Am J Clin Nutr.* Apr;67(4):779S-784S, 1998

Pollitt E, Jacoby E, Cueto S, School breakfast and cognition among nutritionally at-risk children in the Peruvian Andes. *Nutr Rev.* Apr;54(4 Pt 2):S22-6, 1996

Rampersaud GC, Pereira MA, Girard BL, et al, Breakfast habits, nutritional status, body weight, and academic performance in children and adolescents. *J Am Diet Assoc.* May;105(5):743-60, 2005

Riccardi G, Clemente G, Giacco R, Glycemic index of local foods and diets: the Mediterranean experience. *Nutr Rev.* May;61(5 Pt 2):S56-60, 2003

Rizkalla SW, Bellisle F, Slama G, Health benefits of low glycaemic index foods, such as pulses, in diabetic patients and healthy individuals. *Br J Nutr.* Dec;88 Suppl 3:S255-62, 2002

Roberts SB, Pittas AG, The role of glycemic index in type 2 diabetes. *Nutr Clin Care.* May-Sep;6(2):73-8, 2003

Schoenthaler SJ, Bier ID, Young K, et al, The effect of vitamin-mineral supplementation on the intelligence of American schoolchildren: a randomized, double-blind placebo-controlled trial. *J Altern Complement Med.* Feb;6(1):19-29, 2000

Schulz M, Liese AD, Mayer-Davis EJ, et al, Nutritional correlates of dietary glycaemic index: new aspects from a population perspective. *Br J Nutr.* Sep;94(3):397-406, 2005

Sigman M, Whaley SE, Neumann CG, et al, Diet quality affects the playground activities of Kenyan children. *Food Nutr Bull.* Jun;26(2 Suppl 2):S202-12, 2005

Siu PM, Wong SH, Use of the glycemic index: effects on feeding patterns and exercise performance. *J Physiol Anthropol Appl Human Sci.* Jan;23(1):1-6, 2004

Stevenson E, Williams C, Nute M, et al, The effect of the glycemic index of an evening meal on the metabolic responses to a standard high glycemic index breakfast and subsequent exercise in men. *Int J Sport Nutr Exerc Metab.* Jun;15(3):308-22, 2005

Stevenson E, Williams C, Nute M, The influence of the glycaemic index of breakfast and lunch on substrate utilisation during the postprandial periods and subsequent exercise. *Br J Nutr.* Jun;93(6):885-93, 2005

Sunram-Lea SI, Foster JK, Durlach P, et al, Glucose facilitation of cognitive performance in healthy young adults: examination of the influence of fast-duration, time of day and pre-consumption plasma glucose levels. *Psychopharmacology.* Aug;157(1):46-54, 2001

Warren JM, Henry CJ, Simonite V, Low glycemic index breakfasts and reduced food intake in preadolescent children. *Pediatrics.* Nov;112(5):e414, 2003

Wolever TM, The glycemic index: flogging a dead horse? *Diabetes Care.* Mar;20(3):452-6, 1997

Wolever TM, Carbohydrate and the regulation of blood glucose and metabolism. *Nutr Rev.* May;61(5 Pt 2):S40-8, 2003

Wolever TM, Jenkins DJ, Ocana AM, et al, Second-meal effect: low-glycemic-index foods eaten at dinner improve subsequent breakfast glycemic response. *Am J Clin Nutr.* Oct;48(4):1041-7, 1988

Wolever TM, Mehling C, Long-term effect of varying the source or amount of dietary carbohydrate on postprandial plasma glucose, insulin, triacylglycerol, and free fatty acid concentrations in subjects with impaired glucose tolerance. *Am J Clin Nutr.* Mar;77(3):612-21, 2003

Young SN, Clinical nutrition: 3. The fuzzy boundary between nutrition and psychopharmacology. *CMAJ.* Jan 22;166(2):205-9, 2002

CHAPTER SEVEN: Toxins: Part of a Modern Diet

Brighter Water

Azoulay A, Garzon P, Eisenberg MJ, Comparison of the mineral content of tap water and bottled waters. *J Gen Intern Med.* Mar;16(3):168-75, 2001

Brooks BW, Chambliss CK, Stanley JK, et al, Determination of select antidepressants in fish from an effluent-dominated stream. *Environ Toxicol Chem.* Feb;24(2):464-9, 2005

Brooks BW, Foran CM, Richards SM, et al, Aquatic ecotoxicology of fluoxetine. *Toxicol Lett.* May 15;142(3):169-83, 2003

Gauden PA, Szmechtig-Gauden E, et al, Changes of the porous structure of activated carbons applied in a filter bed pilot operation. *J Colloid Interface Sci.* Mar 15;295(2):327-47, 2006

Ritz P, Berrut G, The importance of good hydration for day-to-day health. *Nutr Rev.* Jun; 63(6 Pt 2):S6-13, 2005

Sefcova H, Survey of the microbiological quality of bottled water. *Cent Eur J Public Health.* Feb;6(1):42-4, 1998

Seo GT, Moon CD, Chang SW, et al, Long term operation of high concentration powdered activated carbon membrane bio-reactor for advanced water treatment. *Water Sci Technol.* 50(8):81-7, 2004

Suhr JA, Hall J, Patterson SM, et al, The relation of hydration status to cognitive performance in healthy older adults.: *Int J Psychophysiol.* Jul;53(2):121-5, 2004

Wright JM, Murphy PA, Nieuwenhuijsen MJ, et al, The impact of water consumption, point-of-use filtration and exposure categorization on exposure misclassification of ingested drinking water contaminants. *Sci Total Environ.* Aug 25, 2005

The "Salt Addiction" Theory

Campese VM, Romoff MS, Levitan D, et al, Abnormal relationship between sodium intake and sympathetic nervous system activity in salt-sensitive patients with essential hypertension. *Kidney Int.* Feb;21(2):371-8, 1982

Clark JJ, Bernstein IL, A role for D2 but not D1 dopamine receptors in the cross-sensitization between amphetamine and salt appetite. *Pharmacol Biochem Behav.* Mar 6, 2006

Cooper SJ, Estall LB, Behavioural pharmacology of food, water and salt intake in relation to drug actions at benzodiazepine receptors. *Neurosci Biobehav Rev.* Spring;9(1):5-19, 1985

da Silva RK, Saad WA, Renzi A, et al, Effect of lateral hypothalamus lesions on the water and salt intake, and sodium and urine excretion induced by activation of the median preoptic nucleus in conscious rats. *J Auton Nerv Syst.* Jun 25;53(2-3):195-204, 1995

Davies I, O'Neill PA, McLean KA, et al, Age-associated alterations in thirst and arginine vasopressin in response to a water or sodium load. *Age Ageing.* Mar;24(2):151-9, 1995

De Gobbi JI, Barbosa SP, De Luca LA Jr, et al, Activation of serotonergic 5-HT(1A) receptors in the lateral parabrachial nucleus increases NaCl intake. *Brain Res.* Dec 20;1066(1-2):1-9, 2005

Denton DA, McKinley MJ, Nelson JF, et al, Species differences in the effect of decreased CSF sodium concentration on salt appetite. *J Physiol.* 79(6):499-504, 1984

do Vale CF, Camargo GM, Renzi A, et al, Ibotenate lesion of the medial hypothalamus alters the salt intake and pressor responses to activation of the median preoptic nucleus in rats. *J Physiol Paris.* Feb;91(1):31-7, 1997

Fox J, Guan S, Hymel AA, et al, Dietary Na and Ace inhibition effects on renal tissue angiotensin I and II and ACE activity in rats. *Am J Physiol.* May;262:F902-9, 1992

Jenkins TA, Allen AM, Chai SY, et al, Interactions of angiotensin II with central dopamine. *Adv Exp Med Biol.* 396:93-103, 1996

Lima HR, Cavalcante-Lima HR, Cedraz-Mercez PL, et at, Brain serotonin depletion enhances the sodium appetite induced by sodium depletion or beta-adrenergic stimulation. *An Acad Bras Cienc.* Mar;76(1):85-92, 2004

Lucas LR, Grillo CA, McEwen BS, Involvement of mesolimbic structures in short-term sodium depletion: in situ hybridization and ligand-binding analyses. *Neuroendocrinology.* Jun;77(6):406-15, 2003

Lucas LR, Pompei P, McEwen BS, Salt appetite in salt-replete rats: involvement of mesolimbic structures in deoxycorticosterone-induced salt craving behavior. *Neuroendocrinology.* Jun;71(6):386-95, 2000

Ma FY, Grattan DR, Bobrovskaya L, et al, Angiotensin II regulates tyrosine hydroxylase activity and mRNA expression in rat mediobasal hypothalamic cultures: the role of specific protein kinases. *J Neurochem.* Jul;90(2):431-41, 2004

Oparil S, The sympathetic nervous system in clinical and experimental hypertension. *Kidney Int.* Sept;30(3):437-52, 1986

Parsons LM, Denton D, Egan G, et all, Neuroimaging evidence implicating cerebellum in support of sensory/cognitive processes associated with thirst. *Proc Natl Acad Sci USA.* Feb 29;97(5):2332-6, 2000

Reardon KA, Mendelsohn FA, Chai SY, et al, The angiotensin converting enzyme (ACE) inhibitor, perindopril, modifies the clinical features of Parkinson's disease. *Aust N Z J Med.* Feb;30(1):48-53, 2000

Riggs JE, Neurological manifestations of fluid and electrolyte disturbances. *Neurol Clin.* Aug;7(3): 509-23, 1989

Sakai RR, McEwen BS, Fluharty SJ, et al, The amygdala: site of genomic and nongenomic arousal of aldosterone-induced sodium intake. *Kidney Int.* Apr;57(4):1337-45, 2000

Stancheva S, Alova L, Velkova M, et al, The effects of peptide and nonpeptide antagonists of angiotensin II receptors on the level of brain biogenic monoamines in rats with angiotensin II-induced increase of water intake. *Methods Find Exp Clin Pharmacol.* Jun;24(5):287-90, 2002

Stragier B, Hristova I, Sarre S, et al, In vivo characterization of the angiotensin-(1-7)-induced dopamine and gamma-aminobutyric acid release in the striatum of the rat. *Eur J Neurosci.* Aug;22(3):658-64, 2005

Tanaka J, Hayashi Y, Yamato K, et al, Involvement of serotonergic systems in the lateral parabrachial nucleus in sodium and water intake: a microdialysis study in the rat. *Neurosci Lett.* Feb 26;357(1):41-4, 2004

Turkish S, Cooper SJ, Enhancement of saline consumption by chlordiazepoxide in thirsty rats: antagonism by Ro15-1788. *Pharmacol Biochem Behav.* Jun;20(6):869-73, 1984

van den Buuse M, Zheng TW, Walker LL, et al, Angiotensin-converting enzyme (ACE) interacts with dopaminergic mechanisms in the brain to modulate prepulse inhibition in mice. *Neurosci Lett.* May 20-27;380(1-2):6-11, 2005

Will MJ, Franzblau EB, Kelley AE, Nucleus accumbens mu-opioids regulate intake of a high-fat diet via activation of a distributed brain network. *J Neurosci.* Apr 1;23(7):2882-8, 2003

Yeomans MR, Blundell JE, Leshem M. et al, Palatability: response to nutritional need or need-free stimulation of appetite? *Br J Nutr.* Aug;92 Suppl 1:S3-14, 2004

Zhao X, White R, Huang BS, et al, High salt intake and the brain rennin-angiotensin system in Dahl salt-sensitive rats. *J Hypertens.* Jan;19(1):89-98, 2001

Non-Nutritive Sugars

American Academy of Pediatrics, "Inactive" ingredients in pharmaceutical products: update (subject review). American Academy of Pediatrics Committee on Drugs. *Pediatrics.* Feb;99(2):268-78, 1997

American Dietetic Association, Position of the American Dietetic Association: use of nutritive and nonnutritive sweeteners. *J Am Diet Assoc.* Feb;104(2):255-75, 2004

Butchko HH, Stargel WW, Comer CP, Aspartame: review of safety. *Regul Toxicol Pharmacol.* Apr;35(2 Pt 2):S1-93, 2002 - (conducted in association with The NutraSweet Company)

Dumas TC, Developmental regulation of cognitive abilities: modified composition of a molecular switch turns on associative learning. *Prog Neurobiol.* Jun;76(3):189-211, 2005

Edmundson AB, Manion CV, Treatment of osteoarthritis with aspartame. *Clin Pharmacol Ther.* May;63(5):580-93, 1998

Endres W, Inherited metabolic diseases affecting the carrier. *J Inherit Metab Dis.* Mar;20(1):9-20, 1997

Fernstrom JD, Carbohydrate ingestion and brain serotonin synthesis: relevance to a putative control loop for regulating carbohydrate ingestion, and effects of aspartame consumption. *Appetite.* 11 Suppl 1:35-41, 1988

Fernstrom JD, Branched-chain amino acids and brain function. *J Nutr.* Jun;135(6 Suppl):1539S-46S, 2005

Food and Drug Administration, HHS, Food labeling: health claims; dietary noncariogenic carbohydrate sweeteners and dental caries. Final rule. *Fed Regist.* Mar 29;71(60):15559-64, 2006

Millichap JG, Yee MM, The diet factor in pediatric and adolescent migraine. *Pediatr Neurol.* Jan;28(1):9-15, 2003

Oyama Y, Sakai H, Arata T, et al, Cytotoxic effects of methanol, formaldehyde, and formate on dissociated rat thymocytes: a possibility of aspartame toxicity. *Cell Biol Toxicol.* 18(1):43-50, 2002

Prandota J, Possible pathomechanism of autoimmune hepatitis. *Am J Ther.* Jan-Feb;10(1):51-7, 2003

Sasaki YF, Kawaguchi S, Kamaya A, et al, The comet assay with 8 mouse organs: results with 39 currently used food additives. *Mutat Res.* Aug 26;519(1-2):103-19, 2002

van Os S, Ruitenbeek W, Hopman J, et al, Excitatory amino acid release and electrocortical brain activity after hypoxemia in near-term lambs. *Brain Dev.* Feb 24, 2006

Vermunt SH, Pasman WJ, Schaafsma G, et al, Effects of sugar intake on body weight: a review. *Obes Rev.* May;4(2):91-9, 2003

Weihrauch MR, Diehl V, Artificial sweeteners-do they bear a carcinogenic risk? *Ann Oncol.* Oct;15(10):1460-5, 2004

Yang CR, Chen L, Targeting prefrontal cortical dopamine D1 and N-methyl-D-aspartate receptor interactions in schizophrenia treatment. *Neuroscientist.* Oct;11(5):452-70, 2005

Glutamate

Albensi BC, Ilkanich E, Open-channel blockers of the NMDA receptor complex. *Drug News Perspect.* Nov;17(9):557-62, 2004

Bear MF, Therapeutic implications of the mGluR theory of fragile X mental retardation. *Genes Brain Behav.* Aug;4(6):393-8, 2005

Bhutta AT, Anand KJ, Vulnerability of the developing brain. Brain cellal mechanisms. *Clin Perinatol.* Sep;29(3):357-72, 2002

Cortese BM, Phan KL, The role of glutamate in anxiety and related disorders. *CNS Spectr.* Oct;10(10):820-30, 2005

During MJ, Spencer DD, Extracellular hippocampal glutamate and spontaneous seizure in the conscious human brain. *Lancet.* Jun 26;341(8861):1607-10, 1993

Fisher KN, Turner RA, Pineault G, et al, The postweaning housing environment determines expression of learning deficit associated with neonatal monosodium glutamate (M.S.G.). *Neurotoxicol Teratol.* Sep-Oct;13(5):507-13, 1991

Garlick PJ, Assessment of the safety of glutamine and other amino acids. *J Nutr.* Sep;131(9 Suppl):2556S-61S, 2001

Gillespie CF, Ressler KJ, Emotional learning and glutamate: translational perspectives. *CNS Spectr.* Oct;10(10):831-9, 2005

Halpern BP, Glutamate and the flavor of foods. *J Nutr.* Apr;130(4S Suppl):910S-4S, 2000

Kaneda K, Tachibana Y, Imanishi M, et al, Down-regulation of metabotropic glutamate receptor 1alpha in globus pallidus and substantia nigra of parkinsonian monkeys. *Eur J Neurosci.* Dec;22(12):3241-54, 2005

Kugaya A, Sanacora G, Beyond monoamines: glutamatergic function in mood disorders. *CNS Spectr.* Oct;10(10):808-19, 2005

Lorrin KM, Aboujaoude E, Bullock KD, et al, Double-Blind Treatment With Oral Morphine in treatment-Resistant Obsessive-Compulsive Disorder. *J Clin Psychiatry.* Mar;66(3):353-59, 2005

Martinez F, Castillo J, Rodriguez JR, et al, Neuroexcitatory amino acid levels in plasma and cerebrospinal fluid during migraine attacks. *Cephalalgia.* Apr;13(2):89-93, 1993

Molinuevo JL, Llado A, Rami L, Memantine: targeting glutamate excitotoxicity in Alzheimer's disease and other dementias. *Am J Alzheimers Dis Other Demen.* Mar-Apr;20(2):77-85, 2005

Mutkus L, Aschner JL, Syversen T, et al, Methylmercury alters the in vitro uptake of glutamate in GLAST- and GLT-1-transfected mutant CHO-K1 cells. *Biol Trace Elem Res.* Dec;107(3):231-45, 2005

Niswender CM, Jones CK, Conn PJ, New therapeutic frontiers for metabotropic glutamate receptors. *Curr Top Med Chem.* 5(9):847-57, 2005

Olney JW, Excitotoxins in foods. *Neurotoxicology.* Fall;15(3):535-44, 1994

Olvera-Cortes E, Lopez-Vazquez MA, Beas-Zarate C, et al, Neonatal exposure to monosodium glutamate disrupts place learning ability in adult rats. *Pharmacol Biochem Behav.* Oct;82(2):247-51, 2005

Ritzen A, Mathiesen JM, Thomsen C, Molecular pharmacology and therapeutic prospects of metabotropic glutamate receptor allosteric modulators. *Basic Clin Pharmacol Toxicol.* Oct;97(4):202-13, 2005

Rhodes J, Titherley AC, Norman JA, et al, A survey of the monosodium glutamate content of foods and an estimation of the dietary intake of monosodium glutamate. *Food Addit Contam.* Sep-Oct;8(5):663-72, 1991

Rossom R, Adityanjee, Dysken M, Efficacy and tolerability of memantine in the treatment of dementia. *Am J Geriatr Pharmacother.* Dec;2(4):303-12, 2004

Rundlett KL, Armstrong DW, Evaluation of free D-glutamate in processed foods. *Chirality.* 6(4):277-82, 1994

Sachdev PS, Homocysteine and brain atrophy. *Prog Neuropsychopharmacol Biol Psychiatry.* Sep;29(7):1152-61, 2005

Scopp AL, MSG and hydrolyzed vegetable protein induced headache: review and case studies. *Headache.* Feb;31(2):107-10, 1991

Shipe WD, Wolkenberg SE, Williams DL Jr, Recent advances in positive allosteric modulators of metabotropic glutamate receptors. *Curr Opin Drug Discov Devel.* Jul;8(4):449-57, 2005

Smith JD, Terpening CM, Schmidt SO, et al, Relief of fibromyalgia symptoms following discontinuation of dietary excitotoxins. *Ann Pharmacother.* Jun;35(6):702-6, 2001

Tapiero H, Mathe G, Couvreur P, et al, II. Glutamine and glutamate. *Biomed Pharmacother.* Nov;56(9):446-57, 2002

Tastekin A, Gepdiremen A, Ors R, et al, L-carnitine protects against glutamate- and kainic acid-induced neurotoxicity in cerebellar granular cell culture of rats. *Brain Dev.* Dec;27(8):570-3, 2005

van Os S, Ruitenbeek W, Hopman J, et al, Excitatory amino acid release and electrocortical brain activity after hypoxemia in near-term lambs. *Brain Dev.* Feb 24, 2006

Walker R, The significance of excursions above the ADI. Case study: monosodium glutamate. *Regul Toxicol Pharmacol.* Oct;30(2 Pt 2):S119-21, 1999

Farm Animals on Hormones and Antibiotics

Aarestrup FM, Occurrence, selection and spread of resistance to antimicrobial agents used for growth promotion for food animals in Denmark. *APMIS Suppl.* 101:1-48, 2000

Andersson AM, Skakkebaek NE, Exposure to exogenous estrogens in food: possible impact on human development and health. *Eur J Endocrinol.* Jun;140(6):477-85, 1999

Armstrong JD, Harvey RW, Poore MA, et al, Recombinant bovine somatotropin increases milk yield and calf gain in diverse breeds of beef cattle: associated changes in hormones and indices of metabolism. *J Anim Sci.* Oct;73(10):3051-61, 1995

Aydin H, Onal MZ, Ozkaynak S, et al, Effects of estradiol on cognition evaluated with p300 in in vitro fertilization patients. *Int J Neurosci.* Dec;114(12):1591-9, 2004

Baldwin RS, Williams RD, Terry MK. Zeranol: a review of the metabolism, toxicology, and analytical methods for detection of tissue residues. *Regul Toxicol Pharmacol.* Mar;3(1):9-25, 1983

Berends BR, van den Bogaard AE, van Knapen F, Human health hazards associated with the administration of antimicrobials to slaughter animals. Part I. An assessment of the risks of residues of tetracyclines in pork. *Vet Q.* Jan;23(1):2-10, 2001

Calvert CC, Smith LW, Recycling and degradation of anabolic agents in animal excreta. *Environ Qual Saf Suppl.* (5):203-11, 1976

Davis SR, Gluckman PD, Hart IC, et al, Effects of injecting growth hormone or thyroxine on milk production and blood plasma concentrations of insulin-like growth factors I and II in dairy cows. *J Endocrinol.* Jul;114(1):17-24, 1987

Daxenberger A, Ibarreta D, Meyer HH, Possible health impact of animal oestrogens in food. *Hum Reprod Update.* May-Jun;7(3):340-55, 2001

Eppard PJ, Bentle LA, Violand BN, et al, Comparison of the galactopoietic response to pituitary-derived and recombinant-derived variants of bovine growth hormone. *J Endocrinol.* Jan;132(1):47-56, 1992

Gulay MS, Hayen MJ, Liboni M, et al, Low doses of bovine somatotropin during the transition period and early lactation improves milk yield, efficiency of production, and other physiological responses of Holstein cows. *J Dairy Sci.* Apr;87(4):948-60, 2004

Heitzman RJ, The absorption, distribution and excretion of anabolic agents. *J Anim Sci.* Jul;57(1):233-8, 1983

Hodate K, Ozawa A, Johke T, Effect of a prolonged release formulation of recombinant bovine somatotropin on plasma concentrations of hormones and metabolites, and milk production in dairy cows. *Endocrinol Jpn.* Oct;38(5):527-32, 1991

Hoffmann B, Blietz C, Application of radioimmunoassay (RIA) for the determination of residues of anabolic sex hormones. *J Anim Sci.* Jul;57(1):239-46, 1983

Hoffmann B, Karg H. Metabolic fate of anabolic agents in treated animals and residue levels in their meat. *Environ Qual Saf Suppl.* (5):181-91, 1976

Hogervorst E, De Jager C, Budge M, et al, Serum levels of estradiol and testosterone and performance in different cognitive domains in healthy elderly men and women. *Psychoneuroendocrinology.* Apr;29(3):405-21, 2004

Johnson HD, Li R, Manalu W, et al, Effects of somatotropin on milk yield and physiological responses during summer farm and hot laboratory conditions. *J Dairy Sci.* Apr;74(4):1250-62, 1991

Ganmaa D, Sato A, The possible role of female sex hormones in milk from pregnant cows in the development of breast, ovarian and corpus uteri cancers. *Med Hypotheses.* 65(6):1028-37, 2005

Hegsted DM, Fractures, calcium, and the modern diet. *Am J Clin Nutr.* Nov;74(5):571-3, 2001

Kroes R, Galli C, Munro I, et al, Threshold of toxicological concern for chemical substances present in the diet: a practical tool for assessing the need for toxicity testing. *Food Chem Toxicol.* Feb-Mar;38(2-3):255-312, 2000

Kroes R, Huis in't Veld LG, Schuller PL, Methods for controlling the application of anabolics in farm animals. *Environ Qual Saf Suppl.* (5):192-202, 1976

Kroes R, Kozianowski G, Threshold of toxicological concern (TTC) in food safety assessment. *Toxicol Lett.* Feb 28;127(1-3):43-6, 2002

Lamming GE, Peters AR, Future developments in the manipulation of growth in farm animals. *Vet Rec.* May 23;120(21):495-9, 1987

Leighton JK, Center for Veterinary Medicine's perspective on the beef hormone case. *Vet Clin North Am Food Anim Pract.* Mar;15(1):167-80, 1999

Mader TL, Feedlot medicine and management. Implants. *Vet Clin North Am Food Anim Pract.* Jul;14(2):279-90, 1998

Maki PM, Estrogen effects on the hippocampus and frontal lobes. *Int J Fertil Womens Med.* Mar-Apr;50(2):67-71, 2005

Miller KK, Grieco KA, Klibanski A, Testosterone administration in women with anorexia nervosa. *J Clin Endocrinol Metab.* Mar;90(3):1428-33, 2005

Nesheim MC, Some observations on the effectiveness of anabolic agents in increasing the growth rate of poultry. *Environ Qual Saf Suppl.* (5):110-4, 1976

Neumann F, Pharmacological and endocrinological studies on anabolic agents. *Environ Qual Saf Suppl.* (5):253-64, 1976

Oertel H, Schneider HJ, Stalla GK, et al, The effect of growth hormone substitution on cognitive performance in adult patients with hypopituitarism. *Psychoneuroendocrinology.* Aug;29(7):839-50, 2004

Oomen HA, Schipperijn AJ, Drexhage HA, The prevalence of affective disorder and in particular of a rapid cycling of bipolar disorder in patients with abnormal thyroid function tests. *Clin Endocrinol (Oxf).* Aug;45(2):215-23, 1996

Paige JC, Tollefson L, Miller M, Public health impact on drug residues in animal tissues. *Vet Hum Toxicol.* Jun;39(3):162-9, 1997

Partsch CJ, Sippell WG, Pathogenesis and epidemiology of precocious puberty. Effects of exogenous oestrogens. *Hum Reprod Update.* May-Jun;7(3):292-302, 2001

Rodriguez T, Lavis VR, Meininger JC, et al, Substitution of liothyronine at a 1:5 ratio for a portion of levothyroxine: effect on fatigue, symptoms of depression, and working memory versus treatment with levothyroxine alone. *Endocr Pract.* Jul-Aug;11(4):223-33, 2005

Rumsey TS, Experimental approaches to studying metabolic fate of xenobiotics in food animals. *J Anim Sci.* Jan;56(1):222-34, 1983

Sillence MN, Technologies for the control of fat and lean deposition in livestock. *Vet J.* May;167(3):242-57, 2004

Sone K, Hinago M, Itamoto M, et al, Effects of an androgenic growth promoter 17beta-trenbolone on masculinization of Mosquitofish (Gambusia affinis affinis). *Gen Comp Endocrinol.* Sep 1;143(2):151-60, 2005

Stephany RW, Hormones in meat: different approaches in the EU and in the USA. *APMIS Suppl.* (103):S357-63; discussion S363-4, 2001

Trenkle A, The anabolic effect of estrogens on nitrogen metabolism of growing and finishing cattle and sheep. *Environ Qual Saf Suppl.* (5):79-88, 1976

VanderWal P, General aspects of the effectiveness of anabolic agents in increasing protein production in farm animals, in particular in bull calves. *Environ Qual Saf Suppl.* (5):60-78, 1976

van Leeuwen FX, The approach taken and conclusions reached by the Joint FAO-WHO Expert Committee on Food Additives. *Ann Rech Vet.* 22(3):253-6, 1991

Velle W, Endogenous anabolic agents in farm animals. *Environ Qual Saf Suppl.* (5):159-70, 1976

Vitiello MV, Moe KE, Merriam GR, et al, Growth hormone releasing hormone improves the cognition of healthy older adults. *Neurobiol Aging.* Feb;27(2):318-23, 2006

Wekking EM, Appelhof BC, Fliers E, et al Cognitive functioning and well-being in euthyroid patients on thyroxine replacement therapy for primary hypothyroidism. *Eur J Endocrinol.* Dec;153(6):747-53, 2005

Wilson VS, Lambright C, Ostby J, et al, In vitro and in vivo effects of 17beta-trenbolone: a feedlot effluent contaminant. *Toxicol Sci.* Dec;70(2):202-11, 2002

Zhou J, Zhang H, Cohen RS, et al, Effects of estrogen treatment on expression of brain-derived neurotrophic factor and cAMP response element-binding protein expression and phosphorylation in rat amygdaloid and hippocampal structures. *Neuroendocrinology.* 81(5):294-310, 2005

A Little Ditty about Nitrites and Sulfites

Drew B, Leeuwenburgh C, Aging and the role of reactive nitrogen species. *Ann N Y Acad Sci.* Apr;959:66-81, 2002

Jakszyn P, Agudo A, Ibanez R, et al, Development of a food database of nitrosamines, heterocyclic amines, and polycyclic aromatic hydrocarbons. *J Nutr.* Aug;134(8):2011-4, 2004

Kucukatay V, Savcioglu F, Hacioglu G, et al, Effect of sulfite on cognitive function in normal and sulfite oxidase deficient rats. *Neurotoxicol Teratol.* Jan-Feb;27(1):47-54, 2005

Lester MR, Sulfite sensitivity: significance in human health. *J Am Coll Nutr.* Jun;14(3):229-32, 1995

Wolf OT, Kirschbaum C, Actions of dehydroepiandrosterone and its sulfate in the central nervous system: effects on cognition and emotion in animals and humans. *Brain Res Brain Res Rev.* Nov;30(3):264-88, 1999

Supplements

Boyle P, Severi G, Giles GG, The epidemiology of prostate cancer. *Urol Clin North Am.* May;30(2):209-17, 2003

Cai L, Li XK, Song Y, et al, Essentiality, toxicology and chelation therapy of zinc and copper. *Curr Med Chem.* 12(23):2753-63, 2005

Cameron IL, Munoz J, Barnes CJ, et al, High dietary level of synthetic vitamin E on lipid peroxidation, membrane fatty acid composition and cytotoxicity in breast cancer xenograft and in mouse host tissue. *Cancer Cell Int.* Mar 12;3(1):3, 2003

Frank J, Beyond vitamin E supplementation: an alternative strategy to improve vitamin E status. *J Plant Physiol.* Jul;162(7):834-43, 2005

Leonard SW, Good CK, Gugger ET, et al, Vitamin E bioavailability from fortified breakfast cereal is greater than that from encapsulated supplements. *Am J Clin Nutr.* Jan;79(1):86-92, 2004

Reddy MB, Love M, The impact of food processing on the nutritional quality of vitamins and minerals. *Adv Exp Med Biol.* 459:99-106, 1999

Sabatini S, Ferguson RM, Helderman JH, et al, Drug substitution in transplantation: a National Kidney Foundation White Paper. *Am J Kidney Dis.* Feb;33(2):389-97, 1999

Sandberg AS, Bioavailability of minerals in legumes. *Br J Nutr.* Dec;88 Suppl 3:S281-5, 2002

Shephard GS, Leggott NL, Chromatographic determination of the mycotoxin patulin in fruit and fruit juices. *J Chromatogr A.* Jun 16;882(1-2):17-22, 2000

Schoenthaler SJ, Bier ID, Young K, et al, The effect of vitamin-mineral supplementation on the intelligence of American schoolchildren: a randomized, double-blind placebo-controlled trial. *J Altern Complement Med.* Feb;6(1):19-29, 2000

Sen CK, Khanna S, Roy S, Tocotrienol: the natural vitamin E to defend the nervous system? *Ann N Y Acad Sci.* Dec;1031:127-42, 2004

Shi J, Le Maguer M, Lycopene in tomatoes: chemical and physical properties affected by food processing. *Crit Rev Food Sci Nutr.* Jan;40(1):1-42, 2000

Valko M, Morris H, Cronin MT, Metals, toxicity and oxidative stress. *Curr Med Chem.* 12(10):1161-208, 2005

CHAPTER EIGHT: Immaterial Enrichment for the Brain and Mind

Annesi JJ, Westcott WL, Age as a moderator of relations of physical self-concept and mood changes associated with 10 weeks of programmed exercise in women. *Percept Mot Skills.* Dec;101(3):840-4, 2005

Astin JA, Mind-body therapies for the management of pain. *Clin J Pain.* Jan-Feb;20(1):27-32, 2004

Atran S, Norenzayan A, Religion's evolutionary landscape: counterintuition, commitment, compassion, communion. *Behav Brain Sci.* Dec;27(6):713-30, 2004

Backmand H, Kaprio J, Kujala UM, et al, Physical and psychological functioning of daily living in relation to physical activity. A longitudinal study among former elite male athletes and controls. *Aging Clin Exp Res.* Feb;18(1):40-9, 2006

Berlin AA, Kop WJ, Deuster PA, Depressive mood symptoms and fatigue after exercise withdrawal: the potential role of decreased fitness. *Psychosom Med.* Mar-Apr;68(2):224-30, 2006

Birnbaum L, Adolescent aggression and differentiation of self: guided mindfulness meditation in the service of individuation. *ScientificWorldJournal.* Jun 23;5:478-89, 2005

Blake DT, Byl NN, Mersenich MM, Representation of the hand in the cerebral cortex. *Behav Brain Res.* Sept 20;135(1-2):179-84, 2002

Brown RP, Gerbarg PL, Sudarshan Kriya Yogic breathing in the treatment of stress, anxiety, and depression. Part II-Clinical applications and guidelines. *J Altern Complement Med.* Aug;11(4):711-7, 2005

Bunkers SS, Reflections on the prairie as a creative teaching-learning place. *Nurs Sci Q.* Jan;19(1):25-9, 2006

Callaghan P, Exercise: a neglected intervention in mental health care? *J Psychiatr Ment Health Nurs.* Aug;11(4):476-83, 2004

Chen C, Hardy M, Zhang J, et al, Altered NMDA receptor trafficking contributes to sleep deprivation-induced hippocampal synaptic and cognitive impairments. *Biochem Biophys Res Commun.* Feb 10;340(2):435-40, 2006

Cohen L, Warneke C, Fouladi RT, et al, Psychological adjustment and sleep quality in a randomized trial of the effects of a Tibetan yoga intervention in patients with lymphoma. *Cancer.* May 15;100(10):2253-60, 2004

Colcombe SJ, Kramer AF, McAuley E, et al, Neurocognitive aging and cardiovascular fitness: recent findings and future directions. *J Mol Neurosci.* 24(1):9-14, 2004

Dang-Vu TT, Desseilles M, Peigneux P, et al, A role for sleep in brain plasticity. *Pediatr Rehabil.* Apr-Jun;9(2):98-118, 2006

Davis CJ, Meighan PC, Taishi P, et al, REM sleep deprivation attenuates actin-binding protein cortactin: A link between sleep and hippocampal plasticity. *Neurosci Lett.* Mar 11, 2006

De Moor MH, Beem AL, Stubbe JH, et al, Regular exercise, anxiety, depression and personality: A population-based study. *Prev Med.* Apr;42(4):273-9, 2006

Doran SM, Harvey MT, Horner RH, Sleep and Developmental Disabilities: Assessment, Treatment, and Outcome Measures. *Ment Retard.* Feb;44(1):13-27, 2006

Eggermont L, Swaab D, Luiten P, et al, Exercise, cognition and Alzheimer's disease: More is not necessarily better. *Neurosci Biobehav Rev.* Dec 12, 2005

Erickson KI, Colcombe SJ, Elavsky S, et al, Interactive effects of fitness and hormone treatment on brain health in postmenopausal women. *Neurobiol Aging.* Jan 4, 2006

Ernst C, Olson AK, Pinel JP, et al, Antidepressant effects of exercise: evidence for an adult-neurogenesis hypothesis? *J Psychiatry Neurosci.* Mar;31(2):84-92, 2006

Finucaine A, Mercer SW, An exploratory mixed methods study of the acceptability and effectiveness of mindfulness-based cognitive therapy for patients with active depression and anxiety in primary care. *BMC Psychiatry.* Apr 7;6(1):14, 2006

Galantino ML, Shepard K, Krafft L, et al, The effect of group aerobic exercise and t'ai chi on functional outcomes and quality of life for persons living with acquired immunodeficiency syndrome. *J Altern Complement Med.* Dec;11(6):1085-92, 2005

Galper DI, Trivedi MH, Barlow CE, et al, Inverse association between physical inactivity and mental health in men and women. *Med Sci Sports Exerc.* Jan;38(1):173-8, 2006

Halbower AC, Mark Mahone E, Neuropsychological morbidity linked to childhood sleep-disordered breathing. *Sleep Med Rev.* Apr;10(2):97-107, 2006

Harris AH, Cronkite R, Moos R, Physical activity, exercise coping, and depression in a 10-year cohort study of depressed patients. *J Affect Disord.* Mar 16, 2006

Hill TD, Burdette AM, Angel JL, et al, Religious attendance and cognitive functioning among older Mexican Americans. *J Gerontol B Psychol Sci Soc Sci.* Jan;61(1):P3-9, 2006

Hogan M, Physical and cognitive activity and exercise for older adults: a review. *Int J Aging Hum Dev.* 60(2):95-126, 2005

Kohut ML, McCann DA, Russell DW, et al, Aerobic exercise, but not flexibility/resistance exercise, reduces serum IL-18, CRP, and IL-6 independent of beta-blockers, BMI, and psychosocial factors in older adults. *Brain Behav Immun.* May;20(3):201-9, 2006

Kramer AF, Colcombe SJ, McAuley E, et al, Enhancing brain and cognitive function of older adults through fitness training. *J Mol Neurosci.* 20(3):213-21, 2003

Lai SM, Studenski S, Richards L, et al, Therapeutic exercise and depressive symptoms after stroke. *J Am Geriatr Soc.* Feb;54(2):240-7, 2006

Larson EB, Wang L, Bowen JD, et al, Exercise is associated with reduced risk for incident dementia among persons 65 years of age and older. *Ann Intern Med.* Jan 17;144(2):73-81, 2006

Lou HC, Nowak M, Kjaer TW, The mental self. *Prog Brain Res.* 150:197-204, 2005

Mattson MP, Neuroprotective signaling and the aging brain: take away my food and let me run. *Brain Res.* Dec 15;886(1-2):47-53, 2000

Mattson MP, Duan W, Lee J, et al, Suppression of brain aging and neurodegenerative disorders by dietary restriction and environmental enrichment: molecular mechanisms. *Mech Ageing Dev.* May 31;122(7):757-78, 2001

Mattson MP, Duan W, Wan R, et al, Prophylactic activation of neuroprotective stress response pathways by dietary and behavioral manipulations. *NeuroRx.* Jan;1(1):111-6, 2004

Mattson MP, Wan R, Beneficial effects of intermittent fasting and caloric restriction on the cardiovascular and cerebrovascular systems. *J Nutr Biochem.* Mar;16(3):129-37, 2005

Midtgaard J, Rorth M, Stelter R, et al, The impact of a multidimensional exercise program on self-reported anxiety and depression in cancer patients undergoing chemotherapy: a phase II study. *Palliat Support Care.* Sep;3(3):197-208, 2005

Mikheev M, Mohr C, Afanasiev S, et al, Motor control and cerebral hemispheric specialization in highly qualified judo wrestlers. *Neuropsychologia.* 40(8):1209-19, 2002

Nikolaidis MG, Mougios V, Effects of exercise on the fatty-acid composition of blood and tissue lipids. *Sports Med.* 34(15):1051-76, 2004

Oken BS, Zajdel D, Kishiyama S, et al, Randomized, controlled, six-month trial of yoga in healthy seniors: effects on cognition and quality of life. *Altern Ther Health Med.* Jan-Feb;12(1):40-7, 2006

Ostbye T, Krause KM, Norton MC, et al, Ten dimensions of health and their relationships with overall self-reported health and survival in a predominately religiously active elderly population: the cache county memory study. *J Am Geriatr Soc.* Feb;54(2):199-209, 2006

Pardaens K, Haagdorens L, Van Wambeke P, et al, How relevant are exercise capacity measures for evaluating treatment effects in chronic fatigue syndrome? Results from a prospective, multidisciplinary outcome study. *Clin Rehabil.* Jan;20(1):56-66, 2006

Poudevigne MS, O'Connor PJ, A review of physical activity patterns in pregnant women and their relationship to psychological health. *Sports Med.* 36(1):19-38, 2006

Rogers LQ, Courneya KS, Robbins KT, et al, Physical activity and quality of life in head and neck cancer survivors. *Support Care Cancer.* Mar 15, 2006

Scott JP, McNaughton LR, Polman RC, Effects of sleep deprivation and exercise on cognitive, motor performance and mood. *Physiol Behav.* Feb 28;87(2):396-408, 2006

Shannahoff-Khalsa DS, Patient perspectives: Kundalini yoga meditation techniques for psycho-oncology and as potential therapies for cancer. *Integr Cancer Ther.* Mar;4(1):87-100, 2005

Sharma S, Kaur, Neuroprotective potential of dietary restriction against kainite-induced excitotoxicity in adult male Wistar rats. *Brain res bull.* Nov 30;67(6):482-91, 2005

Shaw FZ, Lee SY, Chiu TH, Modulation of somatosensory evoked potentials during wake-sleep states and spike-wave discharges in the rat. *Sleep.* Mar 1;29(3):285-93, 2006

Siegel DJ, An Interpersonal Neurobiology Approach to Psychotherapy. *Psychiatric Annals.* 36;4, 248-56, 2006

Singh-Manoux A, Hillsdon M, Brunner E, et al, Effects of physical activity on cognitive functioning in middle age: evidence from the Whitehall II prospective cohort study. *Am J Public Health.* Dec;95(12):2252-8, 2005

Song KY, An JD, Premotor and motor reaction time of educable mentally retarded youths in a Taekwondo program. *Percept Mot Skills.* Oct;99(2):711-23, 2004

Tononi G, Cirelli C, Sleep function and synaptic homeostasis. *Sleep Med Rev.* Feb;10(1):49-62, 2006

Vance DE, Wadley VG, Ball KK, et al, The effects of physical activity and sedentary behavior on cognitive health in older adults. *J Aging Phys Act.* Jul;13(3):294-313, 2005

Wachholtz AB, Pargament KI, Is spirituality a critical ingredient of meditation? Comparing the effects of spiritual meditation, secular meditation, and relaxation on spiritual, psychological, cardiac, and pain outcomes. *J Behav Med.* Aug;28(4):369-84, 2005

Waelde LC, Thompson L, Gallagher-Thompson D, A pilot study of a yoga and meditation intervention for dementia caregiver stress. *J Clin Psychol.* Jun;60(6):677-87, 2004

Wall RB, Tai Chi and mindfulness-based stress reduction in a Boston Public Middle School. *J Pediatr Health Care.* Jul-Aug;19(4):230-7, 2005

Weiskopf N, Scharnowski F, Veit R, et al, Self-regulation of local brain activity using real-time functional magnetic resonance imaging (fMRI). *J Physiol Paris.* Jul-Nov;98(4-6):357-73, 2004

Weiss M, Nordlie JW, Siegel EP, Mindfulness-based stress reduction as an adjunct to outpatient psychotherapy. *Psychother Psychosom.* 74(2):108-12, 2005

Williams JM, Duggan DS, Crane C, et al, Mindfulness-based cognitive therapy for prevention of recurrence of suicidal behavior. *J Clin Psychol.* Feb;62(2):201-10, 2006

Woodard FJ, Perceptually oriented hypnosis: cross-cultural perspectives. *Psychol Rep.* Aug;97(1):141-57, 2005

INTERNET ADDRESSES

Preface

Overweight and obesity, adults and children, www.usatoday.com/news/health/2006-04-04-obesity_x.htm

Cost to business, www.academyhealth.org/2005/ppt/florence.ppt

CHAPTER THREE: Brighten Your Mind: Reduce Brain Rust

Skin education, www.skinutrition.net

CHAPTER SIX: Slowly Absorbed Glucose: High-Speed Access to Well-Being

Quinoa pasta, www.quinoa.net

Zone Breakfast Cereal, www.nutritiousliving.com

CHAPTER SEVEN: A Little Toxin Doesn't Hurt

Brita filters, www.shopbrita.com

Espresso makers, www.beveragefactory.com

EPA, www.epa.gov/OGWDW/hfacts.html

Juicers, www.bizrate.com

Magic Bullet Express mixer, www.target.com

Pur water filtration system, www.purwater.com

Seventh century abbott, The Ladder of Divine Ascent, www.TheHTM.org

CHAPTER EIGHT: Immaterial Enrichment for the Brain and Mind

Tryptophan or melatonin, www.herbalremedies.com

Penobscot River, www.blueridgevoyageurs.org/WB_Penobscot.html or www.jackmtn.com/gallery/slideshow.php?set_albumName=eastbranch

CHAPTER NINE

Dark chocolate bar, 1.5 oz, www.godiva.com

Egg fry rings, www.williams-sonoma.com

English muffin rings, www.kitchenniche.ca

Hot dogs, lower in additives and toxins, www.maverickranch.com

Japanese style bread crumbs made of whole wheat, www.iansnaturalfoods.com

Olive oil mister, www.cookscorner.com

Organic olive oil, filtered, www.ecobusinesslinks.com/organic-olive-oil.htm

Organic maple syrup, www.shadymaple.ca

Organic old fashioned oats, www.arrowheadmills.com

Organic stone ground whole wheat flour, www.arrowheadmills.com

Pectin, www.kraftcanada.com

Snuggles hot dog rolls, www. toufayan.com

Stainless steel baking sheets, www.kitchenfantasy.com

Stone ground whole wheat pita, www. toufayan.com

CHAPTER TEN

Psyche Nutrition Sciences, Inc, www.PNSI-Inc.com

Roxiticus Ventures LLC, www.roxiticusventures.com

EKR Therapeutics, www.ekrtx.com

INDEX

A

academic ambitions, 30, 84
addiction:
  definition, 16
  carbohydrate, 71
  cheese, 51, 61
  cheese chips, 85
  chocolate, 63
  cigarette, 12
  cocaine, 12
  fat, 50
  protein, 62
  salt, 79
addictive foods:
  definition, 16
  drive, 16
  fat-laden, 40
  focus, 16
  plasticity, 16
  withdrawal symptoms, 16
addictive drugs:
  cocaine, 14
  definition, 14
  oxycodone, 14
aging, 11
  slowing, 26
aikido, 107
alcohol, 11, 15
aloes, 31
Alzheimer's disease, 24
  antioxidants, 30
  hyperglycemia, 68
American Cancer Society, 87, 92
American Dietetic Association, 84
American Heart Association, 61, 111
amino acids, 13, 53
  branched, 53, 60
  glutamate, 56
  glycine, 57
  phenylalanine, 63, 83
  straight, 54
  tryptophan, 13, 55, 97
  tyrosine, 13, 55
"amnesic eating", 79
anandamide, 63
anger, 18
antibiotic residue in meat, 90
antioxidants, 14
  anthocyanins, 33
  brain cell networking, 39
  "carotenoid", 37
  clean rust, 30
  craving reduction, 19
  "electron-lasers", 30
  flavinoid, 34
  free radical terminators, 30-31
  iced tea, 36-37
  ketchup, 37
  lycopene, 26, 36
  medicinal foods, 19
  neutralize rust, 30
  oleic acid, 45
  phenolics, 34
  polyphenolic, 36
  potatoes, 74
  stone ground wheat, 36
  Table of, 38
  tomato paste, 37
anxiety, 15, 18
  CCK, 57
  exercise, 98
  GABA, 57
  meditation, 105
  prayer, 105
  serotonin, 55
appetite:
  CCK, 57
  endorphins, 57
  olive oil, 22
  suppression, 70, 110
arthritis, 108
artificial sweeteners, 18, 80-85
Atkins, 29, 69
aspartame, 18, 81-84
aspartate, 84
athletes, 10
  zone, 13
Atkins, 29
attention:
  brown-outs, 11
  carbohydrates, 71
  deficit hyperactivity, 15, 20, 103
  EPA, 44
  linoleic acid, 44
  linolenic acid, 44
  meditation, 105
  soy, 59
  tyrosine, 55
avocados, 14, 48, 91
  "fish oil" from, 49

B

behavioral therapy, 101
binge sleeping, 97
"bioavailability", 31, 32
  blueberries, 33
  generic versus brand medicines, 32
  spinach, 33-34
  Sucralose, 84
  tea, 36
  vital oils, 43, 46
bloating, 79
body-building shakes, 60
Body Mass Index (BMI), 99
boredom, 15
brain:
  alarm, 70
  American, 17
  circuits, 10
  corrosion, 11, 27
  fat, 11
  hardware, 6
  "lower", 102
  network, 10
  right side, 8
  rust, 26-29
  software, 6
  toxicity, 24
  upper or executive, 102
  wattage, 11
  -wide web, 13
brain cell:
  aging, 27
  plasticity, 11
  screams, 12
  structure and vital oils, 48
bread, 73
breakfast cereals, 74
breast milk, 87
Bright mocha, 116
BrightFoods:
  "Bioavailable Vital Oils Award", 48
  chef, 146
  chips, 74
  Cookbook, 53, 88, 146
  for Cancer, 60
  fortified peanut butter, 48
  programs:
    business, 149
    food manufacturers, 149
    healthcare, 148
    home, 147
    research and development, 150
    restaurants, 150
    schools, 148
  Pyramid, 36, 61, 151
  smashed potatoes, 75
brown-outs, 11,
  carbohydrates, 70-71
  excitotoxicity, 83
  food, 13
  mood, 11
  thinking, 20

C

caffeine, 63
calcium, 89
calm, 13, 30
calories, 11, 18, 19, 69
  counting, 22
  overload, 29
  restriction, 106

cancer, 11, 18, 19, 22, 69,110
  alcohol, 33
  bladder, 80
  breast, 29, 87
  colon, 29
  lung, 91
  prostate, 29, 74
  skin, 28
  stomach, 61
carbohydrates:
  complex, 65
  glucose, 65
  moderately-absorbed, 65, 156
  "simple", 65
  slowly-absorbed, 13, 72, 155
  rapidly-absorbed, 21, 68, 157
cardiovascular disease, 24
casomorphins, 51
Centers for Disease Control, 21
"cervonic acid", 44
cheese, 18, 51, 61
  "addiction", 51
  glutamate, 56
  phenylethylamine, 51
chest:
  discomfort, 9
cholesterol, 28
cognitive therapy, 101
  hypnosis, 105
  positive imagery, 105
  progressive muscle relaxation, 105
  self-hyper-focusing, 105
concentration, 22
confectioners' sugar, 16
contentment, 16
cooking methods, 29-30
  baking, 29
  barbecuing, 29
  blackening, 14
  broiling, 29
  dark-browning, 14
  frying, 14, 29
corrosion:
  antioxidants, 19
counting-calorie fallacy, 22
crash, 12, 15
  glucose, 69
craving:
  addictive foods, 16, 19
  alarm, 50
  carbohydrate, 65
  definition, 12
  food, 11, 12
  out-of-control, 20
  psychological sugar, 18
  reduction, 19, 20
  salt, 79
creativity, 105
curative medicines, 16
cyclamate, 80
cylinder mills, 35, 36

D

daily protein requirement, 58
Dali lama, 102
daydream, 9
dementia, 20
depression, 9, 15
  aspartame, 82
  GABA, 57
  exercise, 98
DHEA-S, 90
diabetes, 24, 28, 68, 81
diet, 11
  fad, 26
  high calorie, 22
  high-fat, 40
  high protein, 23
  low calorie, 22
  low-carbohydrate, 23
  low-fat, 21
  Mood Diet, The, 59, 159
  pills, 20
  "Sobriety Diet", 59, 159
  wrong-fat, 40
dieting, 20
dimmer switch, 11
disorganized thinking, 15, 21
distraction, 12
DNA, 28, 53, 54, 57, 84
drinks:
  soda, 75
  sports, 75
  Tapple, 75
drug use, 11

E

eating on the run, 111
Edison, Thomas, 98
empty grain, 34-36
energy, 22
  boost, 12
  carbohydrates, 71
  -providing oils, 40
  tyrosine, 55
Environmental Protection Agency, 78
"essential fatty acids", 40
Ester-C, 29
executive thinking, 103
  reward committee, 103
  risk committee, 103
exercise, 11, 13, 23
  aerobic or cardio, 100
  anaerobic or resistance, 101
  cognitive and physical, 106-107
  counseling, 98
  excessive, 100
  physical, 95, 98-101
  push-ups, 99
  spiritual, 95
  trainer, 100
  well-being, 98
exhaustion:
  emotional, 15
  physical, 15
"excitotoxins", 18
  aspartate, 83
  glutamate, 57, 85

F

"Fat Addiction" Theory, The, 50
fatigue, 9, 12
fats:
  bad, 41-42
  good, 21
  ugly, 41
"feeding frenzy", 17, 18
fiber, 34
fidgeting, 9
fire alarm, 8
fish consumption, 63
  school, 152-4
flaxseed oil, 14, 46
flour:
  bleached, 35
  chlorine dioxide, 35
  enriched, 14, 16
  "enrichment", 35
  ransacked, 35
  whole wheat, 16, 73
fluoxetine, 32
focus, 9, 13, 26
  dopamine, 13
food:
  addictive, 16
  consumption accelerant, 79
  convenience, 18
  health and fitness, 30
  heavily processed, 14
  medicinal, 19, 65
  minimally-processed, 14, 20
  over-processed, 16, 21
  unprocessed, 26
food addiction:
  cravings, 12
  hunger, 12
Food Pyramid, 4
  collapse, 21
  reconfigured in 2005, 22
  weak base, 36
formaldehyde, 88
free radicals, 14, 27, 85, 106
  cigarette-smoking, 29
  "corrosive action", 14
  excited oxygen molecules, 26, 27, 29, 30
  iron, 34
  oxidative stress, 29
  ruinous, 20
  terminators, 30-31
  unstable oxygen molecules, 28
"free range", 90

G

glucose, 71
  absorption rates, 155-7
  dips, 67
  is a star, 67
  "pep pills", 68
  rapidly absorbed, 12, 157
  source of energy, 11
  surges, 67
glutamate, 18, 85-87
  cheese, 51
  natural sources, 86
  offset by antioxidants, 85
  seizures, 85
Gold, Mark S., 55
granular sugar, 17
greens, 14
  "fish oil" from, 49
  and vitamin K, 34
grouchy, 9

H

hammer mills, 35, 36
headache, 9, 101
  migraines, 84
head trauma, 11
heart disease, 101
high fructose syrup, 81
Hindus, 53, 108
hormones:
  dairy, 88
  eggs, 89
  meats, 89
  milk, 88
howling hunger pangs, 11
hunger, 12, 18, 22
  alarm, 70
hyper-focusing, 107
hyperactivity, 68
hypersomnia, 96
hypertension, 24
hypnosis, 104, 105

I

ideal weight, 20, 110
  maintenance, 65
  BMI, 99
immigrants, 21
immune system, 29
  aspartame, 81
  exercise, 98
  protein, 53
impatient, 15
inattentiveness, 20
insomnia, 9, 96
insulin, 70
intestinal:
  discomfort, 9, 101
intellectual abilities, 11
  DHA, 44
  EPA, 44
intolerant, 15
iron, 91
irritable bowel syndrome, 18
irritability:
  aspartate, 18
  GABA, 57
  glutamate, 18
  low calorie, 22
  the right brain, 8
  in withdrawal, 15

J

Jonas, Jeffrey, 55
judgmental, 9

K

karate, 107
kata, 107
Keller, Helen, 7
kung fu, 107

L

learning:
  addictive food, 19
  antioxidants, 30
  aspartame, 84
  DHA, 44
  EPA, 44
  gamma linolenic acid, 44
  glucose, 68
  glutamate, 56-57
  hydrogenated fats, 41
  medicinal food, 26
  prayer, 105
  serotonin, 55
  partially hydrogenated fats, 41
  linolenic acid, 44
  the mind, 6
  mood, 6
  sleep, 97
  Sucralose, 84
  trans fats, 41
  saturated fats, 41-42
  tyrosine and, 55
  vital oils, 42, 49
  water, 78
left prefrontal cortex, 8
lifestyle, 95

M

malnutrition, 22, 40
marijuana, 15, 63
medical nutritionist, 21, 38
medicinal foods ratio, 87
meditation, 8, 105-106, 108
memory:
  antioxidants, 30
  arachidonic acid, 44
  aspartame, 84
  corrosion, 11
  DHA, 44
  EPA, 44
  GABA, 57
  gamma linolenic acid, 44
  glucose, 68
  glutamate, 56-57, 85
  linolenic acid, 44
  medicinal food, 26
  saccharin, 80
  serotonin, 55
  sleep, 97
  storing information, 10
  Sucralose, 84
  vital oils, 49
  water, 78
methanol, 84
migraines, 84
mind:
  brain cells, 12
  hunger, 12
  as a learning machine, 6
  "motherboard" of, 6
  muscle-stretching, 107
  sluggishness, 15
  vital oils, 44
mirror cells, 104
mitochondria, 67
monks, 8, 105
  Buddhist, 53
  Orthodox Christian, 53
"more is better", 92
"morphine", 98
MSG, monosodium glutamate, 18, 56
  headache, 18
  irritability, 18
  unnatural sources, 86
mood, 22
  aspartame, 82
  DHA, 44
  EPA, 44
  glucose, 68
  linolenic acid, 44
  meditation, 105
  sleep, 97
  slowly-absorbed carbs, 76
  water, 78
mood swings, 21
moody, 12
motivation and glycine, 57
muscle relaxation, 15, 105
  stiffness, 101
muscles, 10

N

naloxone, 63
nap, 11
neuropsychiatrist, 5
  nutritional, 38, 159, 207
neurotransmitters, 13
  acetylcholine, 13
  adenosine, 57
  CCK (cholecystokinin), 57
  in obesity, 56
  dopamine, 13, 55
  endorphins, 13, 57, 98
  GABA, 57
  instant messengers, 54, 102
  memory, 13
  norepinephrine, 13
  protein, 54
  salt, 80
  serotonin, 13, 55
new brain cells, 10, 20
nicotine fit, 15
nitrates and nitrites, 90
nutritional felony, 36

O

obesity, 21
  BMI, 99
  morbid, 99
  rapidly-absorbed carbs, 68-70
obsessive:
  fretting, 9
  worry, 18
olive oil:
  antioxidant preservatives in, 45
  appetite-suppressing, 22
  endurance, 48
  filtered extra virgin, 14
  "fish oil" from, 49
  glucose absorption, 75
  medicinal food, 19
  not partially hydrogenated, 47
  un-hydrogenated, 45
Onassis, Christina, 78
opiate blockers, 63
Oprah, 49
organic:
  apple juice, 36
  beef, 90
  chocolate milk, 88
  eating, 92-93
  eggs, 90
  farming, 93
  maple syrup, 88
  meats, 90
  milk, 89
  poultry, 90
  spinach, 34
  strawberries, 88
  tomato purees, 37
  wine, 92
osteoporosis, 53, 89
  bone density, 98
"oxidative stress", 27, 90
oxygen:
  deprivation, 11
  in free radical formation, 28
  source of energy, 11
  stimulant, 100
overweight, 21
  BMI, 99
  MA and RA glucose-carbs, 65
overwhelmed, 9
owner's manual, 5

P

pain, 15
  endorphins, 57
panic, 18
  aspartame, 82
partial hydrogenation, 47
  canola oil, 47
  soybean oil, 47
pasta, 73
peace, 105
performance:
  addictive food, 19
  antioxidants, 30
  food, 11
  medicinal food, 26
  sleep, 97
periodic caloric restriction, 106
pessimistic, 9
pesticide residue, 87-88
phenylalanine, 83
phenylethylamine, 63
physical activity, 23
Pilates, 107
pizza, 72
"plaster", 21
plastic, 13, 20
"plasticity":
  definition, 9
  dopamine, 13
  glucose, 67
  meditation, 105
  periodic fasting, 106
  saturated fats, 17
  vital oils, 19, 44
positive emotions:
  electro-chemical activity, 102
  kung fu, 107
  left brain, 8
"positive imagery", 104
pot, 15
power dips:
  hunger, 14
  the mind, 12
  unmanageability, 14
power surges:
  carbohydrates, 71
  the mind, 12
prayer, 105-106
premature death, 21, 24
processed protein:
  canned meats, 59
  cheese, 59
  delicatessen meats, 48, 59
  soy, 48, 56, 60, 86
  whey, 56, 60, 86
"progression", 17
Protein Addiction hypothesis, 63
"Protein Addiction" Theory, The, 62
Prozac, 15, 32, 78
Psyche Nutrition Sciences, 150
psychic space capsule, 15
psychology and biology, 54
puberty, 89

Q

quinoa pasta, 73

R

Rapidly- and Moderately-Absorbed Glucose Addiction Theory, The, 71
red wine, 33
recipes:
  BrightFoods:
    burger buns, 144
    chocolate pecan pancakes, 121
    English muffins, 143
    grain bagels, 128
    grain bread, 120
    grain buns with orange, 145
    grain muffins with banana, 125
    grain wedges with cocoa, 129
    hot dog rolls, 144
    loaf of grain with apple, 123
    mounds of grain with dark chocolate chips, 127
    mounds of grain with oatmeal, 124
    mounds of grain with peanut butter, 226
    pizza, 130-131
    vegan pancakes, 121
  chicken tenders, 138
  chips, 133
  guacamole, 133
  linguini and mini-burgers, 135
  macaroni, broccoli, and cheese, 139
  poultry burgers, 132
  sausage patties, 117
  smashed potatoes, 142
  vegan burgers, 133
  vegan sausage patties, 118
  vegan spheres, 137
  veggie salad, 122
  white chili con carne, 140
  wild rice, corn and cashews, 141
  Yukari dressing, 135

relapse, 102
relaxed, 104
residue in food:
antibiotic, 30
dioxin, 30
hormone, 30
mercury, 30, 78, 152
pesticide, 30, 37
polychlorinated biphenyls (PCBs), 61
Ritalin, 15
"runner's high", 13
Rutgers University, 43

S

saccharin, 80
salt:
"Addiction" Theory, The, 79-80
anxiety, 17
"attack", 79
bloating, 17
convenience food, 21
excess, 17
"feeding frenzy", 17
glutamate, 85
irritability, 17
neurotransmitters, 80
ovarian cramps, 17
snacks, 19
tension, 17
sample menus, 112-115
saturated fats, 14, 17
attention deficit, 17
dim wattage, 23
hangover, 17
hostility, 17
oxidative stress, 28
vital oils, 49-50
senses, 7
shift workers, 98
SIDS (sudden infant death syndrome), 51
sleep, 96-98
adenosine, 57
melatonin, 97
serotonin, 55
tryptophan, 97
sleepfests, 97
seizures, 84, 85
serenity, 104
sluggishness, 21
smart protein, 13, 53-64
organic, 58
percent of calories, 58
tryptophan to serotonin, 55
tyrosine to dopamine, 55
soy, 18, 29, 30
allergies to, 59
"hydrolyzed plant protein", 60
infant formulas, 59, 60
manganese toxicity, 59
spiritual stimulation, 11
Splenda, 70
stem cells, 20
"steroids", 89
stone ground whole wheat, 13, 35, 74
stone mills, 34
stress, 15
exercise, 98
stroke, 24
Sucralose, 84
"sugar high", 12
sugar:
non-nutritive, 80-85
substitutes, 18
swings, 20
sulfites, 90
"Sun Salutation", 108
supplements, 26, 91-92
fish, 30
garlic, 30
lycopene, 37
synapses, 6, 19, 95

T

t'ai chi, 107
Tapple, 36, 74, 116
Teflon, 9
tension:
back, 9
body, 15
neck, 9
Thanksgiving, 13
theobromine, 63
therapist's workplace, 102
thrilled, 13
thunder, 7
toxic, 92
trans fats, 41
ugly fats, 41
"hydrogenation", 41
turmeric, 20

U

USDA, 4, 21

V

Valium, 15
vegan, 29, 53
smart protein, 58
violence, 18
violin players, 10
"virtual reality mini-vacation", 15
"vital oil deficiency", 40
arthritis, 42
Fat Addiction Theory, 50
fatigue, 40
heart attack, 42
immune weakness, 42
learning problems, 40
lupus, 42
memory problems, 43
mood problems, 43
premature aging, 43
sexual dysfunction, 43
skin and hair problems, 40
vital oils, 14
arachidonic acid, 42, 44
daily caloric intake, 43
DHA (docosahexaenoic acid), 42
EPA (eicosapentaenoic acid), 42
functions of, 42-43
gamma linolenic acid, 42
linoleic acid, 40, 44
linolenic acid, 40, 44
oleic acid, 42, 45
right ratio for absorption, 46
Sovereign Seven, 42, 46, 50
vitamin C, 26, 29, 30, 31, 72
vitamin E, 31, 91, 92
"Vitamin F", 40
vitamin K, 34, 90

W

walnuts, 14, 48
"fish oil" from, 49
water, 77-79
contaminants, 158
whale shark, 7
Whole Foods Market, 93
Willis, Thomas, 6
withdrawal, 15
from addictive food, 19
worry, 21

X

Xanax, 50
xenobiotics, 89

Y

yoga, 108

Z

zinc, 91
Zoloft, 78